aging
SMART™

aging
SMART™

Strategies to Live Happier and Healthier Longer

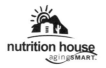

nutrition house
agingSMART.

Proven Advice from Leading Authorities
on Nutrition, Fitness and Mental Health

Library and Archives Canada Cataloguing in Publication Data

Sparks, Carley
Aging Smart: Strategies to live happier and healthier, longer.

ISBN 0-9739799-0-9

Cover design: Angel Guerra/Archetype
Cover photography: Corbis
Text design: Tannice Goddard, Soul Oasis Networking

Nutrition House Canada
80 West Beaver Creek Road, Unit 12
Richmond Hill, Ontario
L4B 1H3

Printed in Canada

10 9 8 7 6 5 4 3 2 1

*This book is dedicated to the memory
of Aldo Domingez and to the
associates of Nutrition House Canada
for their commitment to leading
and fostering well-being, responsibly.*

Contents

Aging Smart

By Carley Sparks — from an interview with
Dr. Theodore Hersh, MD

Aging is a natural and inevitable process. Whether we like it or not, we all grow older, but we are not all affected in the same way. Some fortunate individuals seem resistant to the effects of age. They radiate youthful vitality. Other ill-fated individuals are besieged by time and appear much older than their years. If the years tick by at the same rate for all of us, how can the aging process be so fickle? More importantly, what can we do to keep the effects of time at bay?

To a certain degree, some changes are unavoidable. As the years advance, your hair will grey and eyes dim. Your body will take longer to recover from a hard workout. The odd memory slip or sleepless night becomes more common. These are natural by-products of age.

What is not natural is a disease-riddled, unhealthy body. While it is true that your risk of disease, including cardiovascular disease, cancer and diabetes, the leading causes of death in North America, increases substantially after age 40, this is not an inevitable consequence of growing older. Instead, it is the cumulative effect of years of abuse.

Research shows that lifestyle, not genetics, is the single most important predictor of how we age. It is true that a meaningful connection exists between genetics and aging, particularly in the early decades of life, but as we grow older heredity takes a back seat to our lifestyle choices. According to the landmark MacArthur Foundation Study of Successful Aging, once you enter adulthood your environment and lifestyle account for a full 70 percent of how well you age physically, and 50 percent of how you age mentally! In other words, the ability to improve your health and vitality is largely within your power.

The MacArthur Study also served to identify the top habits of highly successful agers. Among other things, it found that successful agers maintained their physical abilities with exercise, kept their minds sharp with reading, word games, mental puzzles and interesting conversation and stayed actively engaged in life by maintaining relationships with other people and performing productive activities.

Unfortunately, many North Americans are caught in a self-destructive cycle of ill health. Our culture has become synonymous with a high-stress, fast-food lifestyle. We sleep less, eat more and spend more time at work than ever before. Permanently stuck in fast forward, we look for quick fixes and easy solutions — skin products that will erase the lines on our face, drugs to help us sleep at night and miracle diets that promise to shed pounds in a few weeks. In effect, we are doing the precise things that cause premature aging.

The good news is that it's never too late to improve your health. Although it is better to start healthy habits early and sustain them for a lifetime, nature is remarkably forgiving of past health indiscretions. Research shows it is almost never too late to begin healthy habits and, more importantly, to benefit from them. For instance, the risk of heart disease in smokers begins to fall almost as soon as they quit smoking — no matter how long they've smoked — and after five smoke-free years the risk is not much greater than for a person who has never smoked! The same applies to obesity. Being overweight and eating too much fatty food increases the risk of many diseases. But when middle-aged and older men lose ten percent of their body weight, they reduce their risk factors significantly.

You can enjoy optimum health every day of your life and prevent or postpone diseases, provided you start now. And we'll show you how. Aging Smart is about embracing a lifestyle of good health. It is about making the most of your time, the food you eat, the way you exercise and manage your weight; even the way you sleep and deal with stress. It is about enjoying an active and fulfilling sex life and maintaining a sharp mind. More than that, it is about celebrating life!

Before we can understand how to manage each of these areas effectively, we have to start with the question: what causes aging?

Free-Radical Theory

There are many different theories on aging. The one most widely accepted by health authorities is the free-radical theory of aging proposed by Dr. Denham Harman at the University of Nebraska in the mid 1950s. In a nutshell, free radical theory postulates that the aging process is directly related to damage that occurs at the cellular level as a result of various external and environmental influences.

Here's how it works. When oxygen, the body's fuel, is burned or metabolized by cells to perform normal bodily processes, like breathing air or digesting food, by-products called free radicals are produced. These extremely treacherous molecules wreak havoc on the body, damaging healthy cells and vital molecules like lipids, proteins and DNA.

In order to understand free-radical damage, a brief lesson in chemistry is required. All cells in the body are composed of several different types of molecules, which are made up of atoms. To be stable, atoms must have a pair of electrons in their outer orbit. Free radicals are atoms, or groups of atoms, with an odd (unpaired) number of electrons. By nature, such molecules are always looking for a partner to bond with and, in their quest to 'heal' themselves, will literally rip an atom from another molecule (including those in the cell's structure), causing damage to cells and body chemicals. This has a domino effect. When the attracted molecule loses its electron, it too becomes a free radical, beginning a chain reaction.

To make matters worse, free radicals are not just manufactured by the body. Countless more are produced by exposure to sunlight and toxins such as pesticides, tobacco (including secondary smoke and chewing tobacco), excessive alcohol consumption and air pollution. Even fatty meals and heavy exercise, which increases our need for oxygen, produce free radicals.

Many scientists believe that free-radical damage is one of the primary causes of aging and have linked these harmful molecules to more than 50 age-related diseases including cardiovascular disease, immune disorders, neuro-degenerative diseases and a variety of cancers.

What type of diseases free radicals cause depends on the area of the body they attack. For instance, when free radicals take the extra electrons they need from collagen molecules in our skin, the collagen becomes damaged and the skin gets discoloured and looses elasticity. When extra electrons are taken from certain areas of the brain, neuro-degenerative disorders such as Alzheimer's and Parkinson's may result. Likewise, if free radicals borrow electrons from the retinal pigment cells in the eyes, they can cause macular degeneration, the leading cause of blindness in adults.

Antioxidants: Your Natural Defence System

Thankfully, the body has a built-in system of defence against toxic free radicals. Known as antioxidants, these defenders scavenge and neutralize free-radical species by donating the missing molecule and rendering them less toxic (or non-toxic).

Many substances qualify as antioxidants — most vitamins, including A, C and E, several minerals, such as selenium, zinc and manganese, as well as various chemicals found in herbs, fruits and vegetables. Although the body contains a certain quantity of antioxidants in its cells, most are derived from food sources; fruits and vegetables being the most abundant. Usually the more colourful fruits and vegetables, such as the deep orange, yellow, green, red and purple varieties, are the richest sources of antioxidants.

Under normal conditions the body's built-in antioxidant defence system is able to control toxic free radicals and minimize the damage they inflict. But when too many free radicals are produced — due to environmental insults like smoking or excessive time in the sun, coupled with insufficient quantities of fruits and vegetables in the diet — they overwhelm our natural defences and the body goes into a state of oxidative stress.

Unless remedied by increasing antioxidants through diet and supplementation and reducing exposure to toxic substances, the body will slowly break down, leaving it vulnerable to disease.

Key Antioxidants

While there are numerous antioxidants within the body, each of which plays a role in ridding it of excess free radicals, the latest scientific studies reveal two critical points:

1. All antioxidants are not equal
2. Combinations of synergistic antioxidants are far superior to singular antioxidants

The most important synergistic antioxidant is known as glutathione, which acts as 'commander in chief'. Glutathione is found in every cell in the body and is present in most plant and animal tissues from which the bulk of the human diet is derived — fruits, vegetables, liver, meats, fowl and fish. Chicken is very high in GSH content, which may account for chicken soup's legendary medicinal attributes.

Glutathione acts as the body's key antioxidant, detoxificant and protectant. It is the gatekeeper in the respiratory tract and lining of the gut and has multiple functions in disease prevention and in detoxification of chemicals and drugs. The body uses glutathione to preserve the integrity of cell structure and to nullify the effect of toxic free radicals that operate at the cellular level.

Glutathione levels inside the cells must be maintained in order for them to be healthy and have a strong defence system. Without adequate levels of glutathione, cells die, suggesting that glutathione may be a key anti-aging factor. However, glutathione does not work alone.

To provide maximum protection against free radicals, glutathione must work synergistically with other cellular enzymes and antioxidants such as glutathione peroxidase, selenium and vitamins C and E.

It works like this. One antioxidant molecule attacks and neutralizes one free-radical molecule, but in the neutralization process the antioxidant itself becomes oxidized. It then has to undergo a reduction reaction in order to be regenerated as an antioxidant, otherwise it remains as an inert molecule, unable to fulfill its antioxidant function. In some cases, particularly for Vitamin C, the oxidized by-product is itself a toxic free radical and remains so until it is neutralized or regenerated into an antioxidant again.

This is the point where synergy becomes critical. A singular antioxidant cannot regenerate itself. In order to continue to perform its antioxidant function, each oxidized antioxidant must be regenerated by a specific synergistic antioxidant. In the body, glutathione and the mineral selenium (in the form of selenomethionine) assume the pivotal role in this process. In other words, although singular antioxidants such as Vitamin C or Vitamin E are physiologically useful, once they have accomplished their job, attacking a free radical, they are oxidized and become a free radical themselves. However, if they are combined with other specific synergistic antioxidants, particularly glutathione and selenium, they become rejuvenated and then can do their job continuously.

Antioxidants and Aging

As we age, the antioxidant repair process becomes less efficient and is less able to keep up with free radical or oxidative damage, contributing to the development of several age-associated diseases. Scientists are now investigating how diets rich in antioxidants, either from food or supplement sources, can limit the harm caused by oxidative damage and perhaps even slow the aging process. Until more research is available to identify the specific antioxidants for particular diseases, the best way to arm your cellular defence system is by consuming a wide variety of antioxidants found in fruits and vegetables and a synergistic antioxidant supplement, administered in tablets for ease of absorption.

Antioxidant defences are just one small part of the Aging Smart philosophy. Successful aging is a multi-faceted process that envelops every aspect of your life. People who age successfully are healthy, energetic people leading active, vital lives. They don't just want to live longer; like all of us they want to live happier and healthier. And you can too. Improve your overall quality of life by following the nine Aging Smart principles:

- Good Nutrition
- Regular Exercise
- Weight Management
- Skin and Dental Care
- Stress Management
- Good Sleep Habits
- A Healthy Sex Life
- Mental Fitness
- Spirituality

It is not possible to stop aging, but you can significantly slow down the process and prevent or postpone disease. And you may be surprised at how easy it is. It is never too late to start Aging Smart.

Nutrition

By Dr. Joey Shulman, DC, RNCP

Holistic Nutritionist

Carlene, a 39-year-old mother of two, was headed down a dangerous path with her health. A harried lifestyle often did not allow her to eat properly and a 15-year smoking habit was beginning to take a toll on her body. Her weight blossomed from a trim 135 pounds to a stout 160. Her skin was dull and riddled with fine lines around her mouth and eyes. Increasingly she felt bloated after a meal and had regular bouts of constipation. Continuing down this road, Carlene realized she was at high risk of developing cancer and heart disease.

Relationships with food are the hardest to change. Oprah Winfrey, one of the most commercially successful women in the world, battled her weight in public for years before finding a program that worked for her. You should expect too that it will take some work. The good news is that it is never too late to adopt healthy habits and make a significant impact on your health.

Your 40s are a critical time for setting the tone of your health in the years to come. By this time, your body begins to undergo metabolic and physical changes. Your metabolism slows and is less forgiving. Smoking and drinking take a heavier toll on your body. You may find that foods you used to enjoy now disagree with you or cause you to gain weight.

It is also the time when the effects of unhealthy lifestyle choices from your early years begin to rear their heads. The risk of cancer, heart disease and stroke rises dramatically after 40. According to the Canadian Cancer Society, the number of new cases of cancer will increase by an estimated 60 percent over the next 20 years if current trends continue. After age 55, the risk of stroke doubles. For women, coronary heart disease rates rise two to three times after menopause.

While the figures may seem daunting, research shows that prevention of these diseases is directly linked to modified behaviours. One of the most effective means is nutrition. The Heart and Stroke Foundation recognizes that fruits, vegetables, grains and legumes all contain important nutrients, and other cancer-fighting substances called phytochemicals, that strengthen immune function and destroy cancer-causing substances before they do their dirty work. Unfortunately, only 12 to 32 percent of Americans eat the recommended five servings of fruits and vegetables a day. Certain types of fats are also shown to have potent disease fighting qualities but, like produce, tend to be deficient in the North American diet.

In many respects you reach a nutritional crossroads at 40: you can turn your health around and lay the tracks for a happier and healthier life as you age, or continue down a potentially dangerous path toward disease. Experts agree, healthy longevity starts with a healthy diet.

NUTRITION AND THE AGING BODY

As we get older we can expect a number of important changes to take place in our body, metabolically and physiologically.

After age 30, our metabolic rate — the rate at which we burn calories — begins to slow, declining as much as 30 percent over a lifetime. That means you will gain weight if you continue to eat the same way you always have. At the same time, body composition changes. Older adults utilize dietary protein less efficiently, causing lean tissue mass to decrease by as much as 25 percent and body fat to increase. In other words, once firm muscles will become flabby. This is also the time when unhealthy lifestyle choices begin to manifest in various types of health complaints, due to a process known as chronic inflammation.

Digestion

As we age, digestion becomes less efficient due to declining levels of hydrochloric acid (HCl) in the stomach. HCl is necessary for protein digestion and maintains the acid environment of the stomach, which is necessary to prevent bacterial growth. Low HCl levels have been associated with many chronic digestive complaints.

Although common among older adults, digestive complaints are not a normal part of aging. If you experience bloating, indigestion, constipation or diarrhea after a meal, your body is telling you your digestion is off and you need to take care of it.

There are certain nutritional tricks that can help. For one, eat less. In today's fast-paced world we tend to rush through our meals, which leads to over consumption and impaired digestion. Chew your food slowly and drink plenty of fluids with your meals. Secondly, stop eating after seven in the evening. A 12-hour fast is equivalent to a mini-cleanse, helping to step up metabolism while giving the body a chance to repair itself.

Inflammation

Research now indicates that Alzheimer's disease, heart disease, stroke, Parkinson's and arthritic conditions may all begin with an inflammatory process.

Inflammation is the body's first line of defence against harmful invaders such as unwanted bacteria, viruses and a multitude of other health threats. It is what heals and protects the body when you fall off your bike and skin your knee or what helps mend a broken bone. Although this process is critical to maintaining the balance of health, researchers and scientists have now demonstrated that problems arise when the inflammatory process becomes chronic. In fact, hundreds of studies now pinpoint inflammation as the platform from which several disease processes begin.

Unfortunately, the Western lifestyle promotes chronic inflammation. Stress and smoking, combined with a high intake of fast foods and trans fats and a relatively low supply of essential fats and fresh produce, trigger the defence mechanism of inflammation. Because the damage of this process can take years to surface, most people are unaware of the consequences until they become a serious health complaint. With the proper diet rich in anti-inflammatory foods like fruits, vegetables, nuts and fresh fish, chronic inflammation can be prevented and even reversed.

THE THREE NUTRTIONAL KEYS TO HEALTH

Sound nutrition at any age begins with a balanced diet. Unfortunately, many people are confused by what that means. With so many different, and often times conflicting, nutritional strategies advertised — from low-carb to low-fat diets — it can be difficult to discern health fact from health fiction. That need not be the case. Once you understand a few basic principles, it is easy to make sense of nutrition. In fact, there are only three types of food essential to health: carbohydrates, proteins and fats. These are called *macro-nutrients* and should be included in every meal.

Carbohydrates

Carbohydrates are the body's main source of fuel but, like most foods, certain types are better for you than others. Fast carbohydrates, found in refined flour and sugar products, are associated with weight gain, lack of energy, mood fluctuation or mental fogginess. Slow carbohydrates, found in vegetables, most fruits, whole grain breads and legumes, provide a constant source of energy without negative consequences. To optimize digestion, maintain or lose weight and look and feel your best, the key is to consume primarily slow carbohydrates.

To understand the difference between fast and slow carbohydrates you must understand the intricate relationship between blood glucose levels and insulin. Every time we eat carbohydrates, they are broken down into sugar called glucose — the fuel that runs the body. As blood glucose levels rise, they trigger the release of the hormone insulin from the pancreas. One of insulin's many roles in the body is to transport glucose into the cells, to be used as fuel. Once absorbed, glucose levels in the blood are normalized. In this way blood glucose and insulin are in constant communication.

Slow carbohydrates trigger the normal secretion of insulin, helping to maintain blood sugar levels, and provide a constant source of energy for the body. Fast carbohydrates cause an over-secretion of insulin. When this happens, blood sugar levels drop too low and a 'crash' occurs, sending the body into a state of hypoglycemia (low blood sugar). This results in fatigue, moodiness, hunger, mental fogginess and cravings for more carbohydrates. It also causes glucose to be stored as excess fat! In other words, the more refined foods you eat, the more insulin you will secrete. In turn, the more cravings, mood and energy fluctuations you will experience throughout the day, and the more weight you will gain. Excess insulin secretion has also been linked to health problems, such as Type II diabetes, syndrome X (aka metabolic syndrome) and cardiovascular disease.

Foods that tend to be over-secretors of insulin include:

- White sugary foods — candy, pop, cookies, cakes, muffins
- White rice
- White pasta
- White potatoes — baked and mashed
- White bread
- Raisins and dates

- Refined cereal — Kellogg's corn flakes

It is important to remember that insulin secretion is not the enemy. In fact, a normal secretion of insulin as a result of eating a specific food is expected and desired. It is over-secretion of insulin that should be avoided. To determine what levels of insulin secretion different foods cause, refer to the Glycemic Index (GI) and Glycemic Load (GL).

Glycemic Index — The Glycemic Index is a tool that measures the rate at which a food item enters into the bloodstream. The faster the speed of entry, the more insulin will be secreted. For ranking purposes, food is categorized on a scale of 0 to 100, according to its effect on blood sugar levels. The highest measurement is for glucose (GI 100). For the most part, foods that are lowest on the Glycemic Index have the slowest rate of entry into the bloodstream, and therefore have the lowest insulin response. A rating of 55 and below on the Glycemic Index is considered low; 70 and above, high.

To gain all the benefits of eating carbohydrates while avoiding excess insulin secretion, stick to low- to medium-ranked carbohydrates. For the most part, all vegetables (with the exception of white potatoes), most fruits (with the exception of dates, raisins and lychee fruits), whole grains and beans are ranked fairly low on the Glycemic Index. Processed foods such as white bread, white flour, cereals, pretzels, muffins, candy, pop and breakfast bars are ranked higher.

There are several factors that can affect the GI of a food. These include the fibre, protein and fat content of the food, as well as whether it has been cooked or processed.

Fibre, protein and fat act as a brake to lower Glycemic Index ratings. This is why vegetables and fruits, which are high in fibre, and protein-enriched spaghetti have a lower GI rating. This is also why M&Ms candies have a relatively low Glycemic Index rating (GI 41) — they are loaded with fat! The fact that a highly nutritious orange (GI 40) and M&Ms have almost the same Glycemic Index rating highlights an important point. The Glycemic Index rating is an effective tool for measuring only the speed of entry of a food item into the bloodstream — not its health value.

Processing and cooking also affect the GI rating of a food. The refining process pulverizes whole grain foods, thereby eliminating the fibre content (the brake) and enabling the refined flour to rush into the bloodstream very rapidly. This is why a refined piece of white bread has a high GI rating and whole grain, coarse kernel bread has a low GI rating. Simply combining your carbohydrates with proper fat and protein slows down this process, allowing the body to function at an optimal state of health and wellness.

Glycemic Load — Glycemic Load expresses the blood sugar response to specific foods. It tells you how much sugar is in a food, rather than how high it raises blood sugar, by taking into account a food's Glycemic Index rating as well as the amount of carbohydrates it contains per serving. The Glycemic Load of a food is calculated by dividing its Glycemic Index by 100 and then multiplying by its available carbohydrates. A Glycemic Load rating of ten and under is considered low, and a rating of 20 and above is high.

Fast Carbs (High GI Foods)		Slow Carbs (Low GI Foods)	
White plain baguette	95	All-Bran cereal	30
White flour	70	Coarse white kernel bread	41
Wonder enriched white bread	77	Spelt multi-grain bread	54
English muffin	77	Long grain boiled rice	41
Kellogg's Corn Flakes	80	Low-fat fruit yogurt	31
White boiled rice	72	Grapes	46
Puffed rice cakes	82	Apple	34
Raisins	64	Orange	42
Dates	103	Plum	39
Lychee fruit	79	Strawberries	40
Brown rice pasta	92	Chickpeas	31
Stawberry fruit bar	91	Navy beans	38
Jelly beans	80	Lentils	29
Baked potato	85	Protein-enriched spaghetti	27
Instant mashed potatoes	85	Sweet potato	61

Glycemic Load provides important additional information, as Glycemic Index alone can sometimes be misleading. Carrots, for instance, have a relatively high Glycemic Index rating of 71, but have only four grams of total carbohydrates.

$$71 / 100 \text{ x } 4 = 2.84 \text{ GL}$$

Therefore, carrots have a low Glycemic Load rating and will not cause the over-secretion of insulin. White pasta, on the other hand, also has a Glycemic Index rating of 71, but contains 40 grams of carbohydrates.

$$71 / 100 \text{ x } 40 = 28.4 \text{ GL}$$

As you can see, pasta has a high Glycemic Load because it is so dense in carbohydrates. Ideally you want to stick to foods that rank low on the Glycemic Index and have a low Glycemic Load.

Protein

Proteins are the second category of macronutrients, and are an equally necessary part of every diet. In terms of protein consumption, there are two camps that can signal danger. Some people follow the traditional, and outdated, food pyramid that recommends too little protein and too many carbohydrates. Others follow a high-protein diet and are eating an excessive amount of the wrong types of proteins. Both of these approaches can rob internal health and can lead to numerous health problems, including excess weight gain, inflammation, poor complexion, dry skin, fatigue and premature aging. The key to eating protein properly is to consume the right source of lean protein at each and every meal or snack.

Proteins serve many functions in the body. They help maintain proper growth and repair of muscles and tissues. They aid in the manufacturing of hormones, antibodies and enzymes. And they preserve the proper acid-alkali balance in the body. In addition, proteins facilitate the release of the hormone *glucagon*, which has a balancing effect on insulin. This is why adding protein to a meal immediately lowers the secretion of insulin, thereby reducing weight gain.

Unfortunately, due to the surge in high-protein diets, many people are eating excess amounts of the wrong type of protein in an attempt to lose weight. Red meats such as steak, bacon, ribs, cold cuts and hamburgers are typically loaded with artery-clogging and inflammatory saturated fats. These types of fats have been linked to a multitude of disease processes including heart disease, stroke, high blood pressure, cancer and hormonal disturbances in both men and women.

Lean proteins, on the other hand, deliver all the benefits of protein without the health risks and should be included in your daily diet. These include:

- Lean turkey or chicken breast
- Fish such as wild salmon, tuna (use sparingly and use light, not white, tuna as it is lower in mercury content), sole, cod, clams, oysters, mackerel, haddock, halibut, crab, lobster, sardines, sea bass, shrimp, trout (fresh-water), tilapia and scallops
- Egg whites and omega-3 eggs
- Low-fat yogurt
- Skim milk
- Low-fat cottage cheese or other low-fat cheeses
- Goat cheese
- Protein powder
- Tofu: veggie burgers, imitation ground beef, seasoned firm tofu in a stir-fry
- Soy cheese
- Soymilk
- Tempeh (soybean cake with a smoky, nutty flavor. It can be marinated or grilled and added to stir-fries, casseroles and chili)
- Occasional lean beef or pork

On average, women require 70 to 90 grams of protein per day; men, 100 to 120 grams. As a guideline, a 115-gram piece of chicken or fish equals approximately 28 grams of protein. Eighty-five grams of sirloin steak or one scoop of protein powder yields about 25 grams of protein. Thirty grams of low-fat cheese is the equivalent of seven grams. The palm of your hand, minus your thumb and fingers, or a deck of cards equals an 85-gram serving of fish or meat. Vegetable sources are considerably lower in protein. One cup of lima beans provides approximately 15 grams of protein, and 115 grams of tofu about ten grams.

Fats

Fat is the third type of macronutrient the body relies on to run smoothly. In fact certain types of 'good' fats are so critical to the functioning of our system that without them our health would instantly suffer. The key is to emphasize 'good' fats and avoid 'bad' fats.

There are five categories of fats:

1. trans fatty acids — the 'very bad' fats
2. saturated fats — the 'bad' fats
3. polyunsaturated fats — the 'so-so' fats
4. monounsaturated fats — the 'good' fats
5. essential fats — the 'very good' fats

Trans fatty acids — Trans fatty acids are found in numerous foods on our grocery store shelves, including commercially packaged cookies and crackers, and commercially fried food such as french fries, microwaved popcorn, vegetable shortening and some margarines. These fats are created when technologists alter the chemical structure of a polyunsaturated fat (i.e. vegetable oil) from a round shape to a straight chain. Known as *hydrogenation*, this process results in a synthetic fat that is shown to cause plaque buildup in arteries, increase cholesterol levels, promote cancer and increase the risk of cardiovascular disease. In addition, due to their shape, trans fatty acids are extremely difficult for the body to get rid of.

To determine how much trans fat is in the products you buy, check the label under the Total Fat section. Ideally, you want to eat as little trans fat as possible, and certainly no more than three grams per day. It should be noted that under the FDA regulations, if a product contains less than 0.5 grams of trans fat, it may be declared as zero. If you eat three to four servings of an item, you could be eating as much as two grams of trans fat. If the amount of trans fat is not listed, simply add up the values for saturated, polyunsaturated and monounsaturated fats. If the number is less than the "total fats" shown on the label, the unaccounted fat is derived from trans fat. Alternatively, look for the words "hydrogenated" or "partially hydrogenated," which indicate the product contains trans fatty acids.

Saturated fats — Saturated fats are found in animal products such as butter, cheese, whole milk, ice cream and cream. They are also found in fatty meats and in some vegetable oils such as coconut, palm and palm kernel oils. Usually solid, or almost solid, at room temperature, saturated fats are 'bad' fats because they make the body produce more cholesterol and, when consumed in excess, can raise the level of 'bad' cholesterol known as *low density lipoprotein* (LDL). High LDL levels (above 160 mg/dl) increase heart disease risk. In addition to raising LDL levels, research has demonstrated that eating too many of the wrong fats such as saturated and trans fatty acids increases inflammation.

When looking at a food label, pay very close attention to the percentage of saturated fat and avoid or limit any foods that are high (over 20 percent saturated fat). Saturated fats should be kept to five percent or less of total dietary fat intake.

Polyunsaturated fats — Polyunsaturated fat remains liquid at room temperature and is found in vegetable oils made from safflowers, corn, sunflowers and soybeans. Although polyunsaturated fat lowers the level of the 'bad' cholesterol lipid LDL, it is also believed to lower the 'good' cholesterol lipid known as high-density lipoprotein (HDL).

Monounsaturated fats — These 'good' fats are found in olive, canola and peanut oils, and in avocados. These fats appear to lower 'bad' LDL cholesterol and have minimal or no effect on the 'good' HDL cholesterol. Olive oil contains the highest amount of monounsaturated fats of all the edible oils. The best type of olive oil is labeled "extra virgin," and made from the first pressing of the olives. This oil is very flavorful and can be used for cooking or in salad dressings.

Essential fats — Essential fatty acids are vital for health and cannot be produced by the body. Every living cell in the body needs essential fatty acids to rebuild and produce new cells. There are two basic categories of essential fatty acids: omega-3 fatty acids and omega-6 fatty acids.

The ideal ratio of omega-6 to omega-3 is approximately 1:1. However, due to the over consumption of processed foods and of safflower and sunflower oils, most North Americans are chronically deficient in omega-3 essential fats. The average ratio ranges between 20:1 and 30:1. This creates an imbalance. When too many omega-6 fats are consumed, the body becomes deficient in omega-3 fats. Allergies, eczema, inflammatory conditions (i.e. arthritis), constipation, dry skin and premature aging have all been linked to a deficiency of this precious fat.

Optimal omega-3 food sources are flaxseed oil, omega-3 eggs, deepwater fish and fish oil, walnuts and walnut oil and soybeans. Optimal sources of omega-6 are those found in raw nuts, seeds, legumes, borage oil, grapeseed oil and primrose oil.

EATING SMART

Now that you understand the fundamental principles of digestion and nutrition — slow carbohydrates, lean protein and 'good' fats — it is easy to adjust your eating habits. Simply incorporate the three macronutrients — protein, carbohydrates and fats — into every meal and you will have a balanced diet that provides variety and flexibility. You will keep your metabolism revved, your energy up and your immune system strong. You will get the proper phytochemicals (plant chemicals) in your diet and enough of the 'good' fats that will keep your skin, hair and nails looking their best.

The optimal breakdown of food for each meal should roughly fall into:

- 40 percent of calories derived from slow carbohydrates
- 30 percent of calories derived from lean proteins
- 30 percent of calories derived from essential fats

It is important to note that fats are considerably more dense in calories. Use fat conservatively by sprinkling nuts

on a salad, using oil in a salad dressing or adding a spoon-
ful of flaxseed oil to a morning shake. If you're eating nuts,
have half a handful per meal or snack.

Supplements for Optimal Nutrition
Although your focus should be on eating foods that will
provide you with the nutrition you need to keep your body
strong and functioning optimally, even the most vigilant
people will have trouble at times. When you are too rushed
to eat properly, strategic supplements can help ensure you
are meeting your nutrient goals.

Multivitamins — In 2002, the *Journal of the American
Medical Association* reversed its stance on nutritional
supplements and published a study recommending that
all adults take a daily multivitamin. The key is choosing a
high quality multivitamin/mineral. Look for a multivitamin
supplement that contains standardized extracts and has an
expiration date, quality assurances, and company contact
information.

For optimal absorption, always take your multivitamin
with food. Do not take your multivitamin with coffee. Coffee
is too acidic and can destroy some of the bioavailability of
certain nutrients. It is important to note multivitamins are
not a license to eat poorly, but rather a nutritional safety
net for when we don't always eat optimally.

Fish oil — Fish oil is a rich source of the omega-3 fatty
acids eicosapentaenoic acid (EPA) and docosahexaenoic acid
(DHA). Of the numerous roles they play in the body, these
precious fats have been shown to help protect against,
and even reverse, the ill effects of a vast number of health

conditions, including heart disease, high cholesterol, high blood pressure, breast cancer and depression. EPA and DHA also have anti-inflammatory activity and are used to prevent and treat various inflammatory conditions, such as Crohn's disease and rheumatoid arthritis.

Purchase a fish oil that has been distilled for purity, is enteric coated and has a significant percentage of EPA and DHA (at least 30 percent). Store fish oil supplements in the fridge after they have been opened, to preserve freshness, and always take with food.

Probiotics — Probiotics are beneficial bacteria that are critical to good digestive health. Research has suggested that probiotic bacteria help reduce the risk of certain intestinal illnesses, including diarrhea, irritable bowel disease, Crohn's and colitis. In addition, probiotics assist lactose intolerant people with lactose digestion and enhance the immune function.

Most probiotic products contain bacteria from the genera *Lactobacillus* or *Bifidobacterium*, two normal inhabitants of the healthy intestine. Look for a product that offers a mix of strains and provides a minimum of two billion organisms per capsule.

Fitness

By Mike Demeter, BPHE, CSCS, CFA Kin, Specialist CMT
Senior Trainer, GoodLife Fitness Centre

> *Jim, an industrial electrician, was 40 pounds over-weight and increasingly unhappy with the way he looked. Unable to keep up with his active wife or the demands of his job, his quality of life deteriorated with each passing year. He questioned whether his spouse still found him attractive, and doubted his acceptance by family and peers. At 50 years of age, Jim realized that unless he started making changes in the way he looked and felt, every aspect of his life would suffer.*

Physical fitness is arguably the most important aspect of living. It is what enables you to interact meaningfully with the world, and what determines your ability to function independently. With age, fitness levels naturally decline and physical infirmities begin to surface. Things that you never had difficulty with before become problematic — you may find it hard to tie your shoes or open jars. If, like Jim, you are not fit enough to keep up with your mate, your children or the demands of your job, your relationships and outlook on life will inevitably suffer.

More than any other aspect of health, fitness is tied to self-esteem. How we look has a tremendous impact on how we feel. When you are dissatisfied with what you see in the mirror, it affects the way you present yourself to the world and the way you interpret how other people view you. In a personal relationship, intimacy issues may result from poor body image. You may not want to undress in front of your partner or be naked during intercourse, for fear of rejection. In work and life, esteem issues may prevent you from accomplishing your goals and are often what keep people from joining a gym. There is a misconception that the gym is a place for the beautiful people. In reality, if you take the cast of Cheers and put them in spandex you would have a more accurate reflection of the gamut of people who frequent fitness centres.

Of course, not all people will feel the effects of being unfit to the same degree. The desire to improve physical fitness may simply stem from a recent doctor's test or the desire to look and feel better. Whatever your motivation, the benefits are numerous. In addition to boosting strength and energy levels, exercise is shown to mitigate the aging process by improving mood, thwarting disease and preventing injury. Even modest improvements yield significant pay offs.

The key to success is developing a program that caters to your specific needs and goals. You may be surprised to see that there are no exercise recommendations in this chapter. Cookie cutter programs are written for the general masses, and do not take into consideration the specific ability level and limitations of the individual or the training modalities best suited to him or her. Simply put, these systems are not the ideal way to improve your physical fitness.

Instead, we offer a strategy for approaching physical fitness. The advice in this chapter is based on the assumption that you will consult a fitness expert, in the form of an exercise class leader, personal trainer or gym employee. Before you say you cannot justify the expense of a personal trainer, consider this: we use professionals for everything from fixing our car to cutting our hair. Why is it we feel that a magazine or a video is all that is required to tell us what to do at the gym? If our longevity and happiness lies in our health, it follows that we deserve educated advice when undertaking a fitness program.

FITNESS AT 40 AND BEYOND

Your fitness level at 40 will not be what it was at 25, nor will your body be as forgiving as it once was to the rigors of exercise or to unhealthy lifestyle choices — poor diet, high stress, inadequate sleep. As we get older, hormone levels decline and our ability to function physically becomes impaired. Some men will begin showing signs of andropause — fatigue, loss of strength, low energy, poor concentration, irritability, decreased interest in sex — due to declining testosterone levels — and will have difficulty building and maintaining muscle mass. For women, perimenopause and menopause become concerns. With declining estrogen levels, bone density and muscle mass can drop off, while 'bad' cholesterol levels and fat increase. Many of these symptoms can be controlled, and even reversed, with regular exercise, resulting in a younger looking and happier version of you.

Benefits of Exercise

Regular exercise is an integral part of an Aging Smart program. Among its numerous benefits, exercise improves stamina and mood, wards off disease and even increases life span. It is important to note that exercise is only one part of the Aging Smart equation. Without proper nutrition, sleep and stress management, exercise will have the opposite effect. Subjecting an exhausted body to a workout will make you prematurely old. As fitness columnist Chris Shugart points out, "You can't out-train a bad diet."

Best of all, it is never too late to start turning back the clock. A Harvard study demonstrated that nursing home patients aged 87 to 90 years gained muscle, strength and bone density when put on a weight-lifting program. Here are a few of the ways exercise helps you to age smart:

Mood — Improved mood is a pleasant side effect of exercise. A study out of the University of Texas showed that just 30 minutes of brisk walking can immediately boost the mood of depressed patients, delivering the same quick pick-me-up as people get from cigarettes, caffeine or binge eating.

Mental acuity — Increasing physical activity is shown to decrease cognitive decline. A recent British study showed that busy professionals who exercise during the day feel more productive and are less likely to spout off at colleagues and slam down the phone after they've worked up a sweat. In the study, six out of ten workers said their time management skills, mental performance and ability to meet deadlines improved on days when they exercised, amounting to a 15 percent boost in overall performance. The type of exercise did not seem to matter.

Disease risk — Vigorous activity that raises the heart rate can protect against heart attacks and other cardiovascular conditions, the leading cause of mortality in North America, by burning calories, lowering blood pressure and improving metabolism. It may also reduce the risk of diabetes.

Bone density — Weight-bearing exercises are shown to help maintain and increase bone density, thereby reducing the risk of osteoporosis and bone fractures. Even moderate programs yield benefits. Researchers at Johns Hopkins determined that for people aged 55 to 75 a moderate program of physical exercise generally maintains bone mass and, in some cases, offers modest improvements. Those who exercised hardest and showed the greatest increases in aerobic fitness, muscle strength and muscle tissue demonstrated the highest gains in bone mass.

Longevity — Exercise may extend life. A Harvard Alumni study showed that previously sedentary men who began exercising after the age of 45 enjoyed a 24 percent lower death rate than their classmates who remained inactive.

Strength — Strength becomes increasingly important as you age, and by your 70s and 80s it is central to your quality of life. Your ability to get in and out of bed and the bathtub, to cook and get dressed will ultimately determine whether you are able to live independently or require assistance.

Although it is never too late to start developing muscle strength, the earlier you start, the more significant the benefits.

Energy — Working out actually gives you more energy. In fact, the more vigorous the activity, the greater the energy reward. One study found that middle-aged women who lifted weights for a year became 27 percent more active in daily life than before they started strength training.

STRATEGIZING FOR SUCCESS

By now you may be inspired to get in shape. You are probably thinking about the exercises or programs you did in the past — which ones you liked and those that you didn't — and may even be thinking about getting started on one as early as tomorrow. Wait!

Taking a haphazard approach to fitness is a sure fire way to set yourself up for failure. If you have tried to get fit in the past — by taking up jogging or heading to the gym to pick up where you left off many months or years ago — you know that you returned home with stiff, over-worked muscles and were in fact worse off than when you walked through the doors. I call this the "Ready, Fire, Aim" approach. It is not a recipe for success.

To succeed in the long term you need a fitness strategy with clearly defined goals and a map of how to accomplish them. A successful strategy is also mindful of the risk factors you will have to work around, and evolves as your fitness level improves. What is right for you on day one of your fitness program will have changed by day 30, and by the end of the year will have evolved completely.

Stage One: Needs

Needs are the things that keep you alive, vibrant and healthy. In the rat race of life, we all want to keep up with 'traffic' no matter what our age. By the time you are 40 or 50, your body has been driven hard to keep up, and will likely be in need of repair before you start pushing it past its current performance levels. Just as you would have a diagnostic exam performed on your car before deciding what repairs to undertake, you must accurately assess the current condition of your body before undertaking a fitness regime.

In fitness, this is accomplished with what is called a PAR-Q: Physical Activity Readiness Questionnaire. Developed by Health Canada, the PAR-Q assesses health risk factors, such as high blood pressure, light headedness and bone or joint problems, to identify the small number of adults for whom physical activity might be inappropriate.

Physical Activity Readiness Questionnaire

1. Has your doctor ever said you have heart trouble?
2. Do you frequently have pains in your heart and chest?
3. Do you often feel faint or have spells of severe dizziness?
4. Has a doctor ever said your blood pressure was too high?
5. Has your doctor ever told you that you have a bone or joint problem such as arthritis that has been, or might be, aggravated by exercise?
6. Is there a good physical reason not mentioned here why you should not follow an activity program even if you wanted to?
7. Are you over age 65 and not accustomed to vigorous exercise?

If you answered yes to one or more of these questions, it is recommended that you consult your doctor prior to increasing your physical activity or taking a fitness test. Even if you didn't, it is a good idea to visit your health practitioner(s) for a blood chemistry profile and chiropractic alignment analysis prior to embarking on a fitness regime. The PAR-Q only takes into account serious health threats. It does not factor in non-critical risk factors that could put you in harm's way. If, for instance, you always carry your bag on one shoulder, your spinal column will likely be out of alignment. At the gym, this will affect your ability to use proper technique when performing specific movements, such as a chest press, causing you to develop the wrong muscle groups while trying to do the 'right' movements. Or there may be blood chemistry problems you are unaware of. Men who have a short fuse or attention span, or find themselves crying during Bell commercials, probably have low testosterone levels, and no matter how hard they work out will have a hard time maintaining muscle mass. Your doctor and chiropractor can identify these types of problems before you make them worse.

Stage Two: Goals

As soon as you understand your needs, you can start establishing your goals. Most likely you have a pretty clear idea of what you want to accomplish — weight loss or gain, improved energy levels, better stamina etc. But for your goals to have meaning you have to establish the reason behind them. Ultimately this will be your motivational positioning statement. If you want to lose weight, for instance, consider why that is important to you, beyond simply looking better. Perhaps you want to fit into your favourite red dress or, like Jim, you may want to keep up with your spouse or children. If you consider weight loss as one way to recapture the way you felt in your youth, or as a way to maintain a happy and fulfilling relationship with your significant other(s), you will be much more inspired to stick with your fitness program than by the general goal of dropping a few pounds.

At the same time, be realistic about what fitness will do for you. For most people, getting fit is about self-esteem as well as being a cosmetic endeavour. They feel as though the void in their happiness could be cured by becoming more attractive. When they start closing in on their goal and discover that the gym alone won't do it — they still suffer poor self image, or question their attractiveness and acceptance by family and peers — the sabotage begins. They start making poor decisions. Improving your fitness is a step towards feeling better, but it is not a solution in itself.

Having established your purpose, you can help yourself stick with your goals by establishing a 'Win Box'. Focus on your accomplishments, no matter how insignificant they may be. In this way you can ensure that you are pursuing tangible goals.

Stage Three: Mapping your Path to Fitness
Once you have been assessed physically and have clearly defined your goals, your personal trainer can plan a fitness regime that will get you there as quickly and efficiently as possible. A good trainer will recommend a program that takes into consideration your lifestyle and appeals to your interests as well as your goals.

Be honest about what you can stick with. Getting fit may mean a few adjustments in your lifestyle, but it does not mean forsaking normal living. Explain to your trainer what you are, and are not, prepared to give up. By following the 80/20 rule — investing in good health 80 percent of the time and indulging 20 percent of the time — you can offset the negative effects of less healthy choices by adding in positive elements. For instance, you do not have to give up wine with dinner if you are prepared to cut back to two glasses a night and start your meal with a protein shake.

Once you have agreed on a plan, stay within the parameters given to you. Some people extend their workout, thinking they will reap more benefits, and end up hurting themselves. A 40-minute run after a weight training session will more than likely put you at risk of damaging a knee or ankle, and in the end will put you behind in your fitness schedule.

FITNESS FUNDAMENTALS

Exercise, done correctly, is a controlled exertion based on an ongoing process. As you accomplish one fitness goal you turn your attention to another, evolving to higher levels of functioning. While there are numerous ways to approach physical fitness, there are really only a few simple goals. We are born with the ability for primal movement patterns — push/pull, twist and squat — coupled with the ability to maintain a steady gait. It is these features that we want to preserve and optimize with resistance training — to maintain strong muscles and bones — with aerobic exercise — to condition the cardiovascular system — and with flexibility training — to ensure strength and suppleness.

Resistance Training

Resistance training (i.e. weight lifting) builds lean muscle mass, boosting your metabolism and promoting loss of body fat. The more muscle you have, the more calories you burn. One pound of muscle burns roughly 50 calories per day, compared to one pound of fat, which burns only two to three calories per day. In fact, resistance training plays an even stronger role in weight loss than aerobic activity.

Resistance training is particularly important for adults. In your 40s you will notice the undesirable shift in body composition that happens with age. We start to lose our muscle mass and gradually gain body fat, especially around the mid-section. Resistance training helps slow down muscle loss and improves balance, endurance and bone density, reducing the risk of osteoporosis. Contrary to popular belief, women do not get 'big' from weight training. Resistance training will tone muscles. It does not result in the bulky muscles of female body builders, which may have been augmented with hormones and steroids.

There are approximately two to three exercises for every muscle in the body; everything beyond that is a variation. The bicep can raise the arm or flex the elbow. Adding a twist, weights, resistance or other variance simply increases the stress curve. A good resistance training program alternates muscle groups, and provides constant change to prevent injury, such as carpal tunnel, caused by repetitive movements.

Aerobic Activity

Aerobic activity that raises the heart rate helps keep your cardiovascular system fit, and associated diseases at bay.

It can also burn calories, lower blood pressure, improve metabolism, enhance sleep and boost your mood.

When it comes to aerobic training, it is the intensity of your effort that counts. Long, drawn out cardiovascular training done too often is degenerative. In fact, marathon runners, who are often considered the picture of good health, have the highest level of degenerative conditions. A good cardiovascular training program incorporates progressive resistance followed by adequate rest, nutrition and hydration. If you can walk half a mile now, increase your speed one tenth of a mile at a time until you can jog, run and then sprint that half mile.

Flexibility

A study by the Buck Institute on Aging suggests that imbalance-related falls may become the number one cause of disability in baby boomers when they reach their 80s, ahead of arthritis, heart disease and dementia.

The most effective way to maintain balance and flexibility is a stretching program. Stretching releases muscle tension, improving posture. It strengthens lower back muscles, minimizing back problems. And it protects against injury and soreness. A good stretching program targets all of the major muscle groups, and should be performed after every workout. In some cases, your resistance training program will incorporate a number of the stretches you need.

A typical healthy week includes a balance of all three elements: three 20-minute sessions of resistance training, two 40-minute sessions of cardiovascular activity and active stretching after every workout once the body is warm. For example, you may weight train on Monday, Wednesday and Friday, focusing on different patterns and stretching each time. Swim on Tuesday. Do an aerobic dance class on Thursday. And go window shopping or park walking on the weekend. The key is to keep at your program and make fitness part of your everyday life. In the words of Coach Charles Stayley, "Average people who do the right things get better results than brilliant people who do the wrong things."

Weight Management

By Sherry Torkos, BScPharm

Pharmacist, Author, Certified Fitness Instructor

Rhonda, a 46-year-old housewife, was 30 pounds over-weight and constantly tired. Over the years she had tried just about every fad diet, but inevitably always seemed to gain the weight back. Determined to lose weight, she reduced her caloric intake to 1,500 calories a day and joined the local gym. But, despite her efforts, her weight would not budge.

If you are struggling with your weight like Rhonda, you have plenty of company. Currently in the United States, over 60 percent of adults are overweight, and one-quarter are classified as obese. In Canada, the figures are equally dire. Approximately 48 percent of Canadian adults carry excess poundage and 15 percent are obese, according to the 2000/2001 Canadian Community Health Survey.

Obesity has reached epidemic proportions in North America. And we are paying for it with our health, our happiness and our pocket book. Not only is being overweight a risk factor for many chronic diseases, such as diabetes, heart disease and certain cancers, it also has far-reaching effects on a person's self-esteem and confidence. Together these afflictions are costing the health care system an estimated $117 billion per year in the United States alone.

What is clear is that the fad diets and weight-loss gimmicks are not working. Despite the fact that Americans spend more than $33 billion annually on weight-reduction products, such as diet foods and drinks, the rate of obesity has increased by more than 60 percent over the last ten years. And the future doesn't look any slimmer. Even when dieters do lose weight, research shows that most (66 percent) will gain it back within a year, and 97 percent within five years.

The fact is weight loss is a much more complex topic than once believed, and is not going to be resolved by a magic pill, formula or machine. Old beliefs about calorie restriction are being replaced by a better understanding of calorie quality, and an increased awareness of the impact of other health factors, such as thyroid dysfunction and hormone imbalances. Health authorities agree that, in order to maintain long-term weight loss, you need to make long-term changes to your lifestyle.

DEFINING OBESITY

There are a variety of methods used to determine whether you are carrying excess weight and are at risk of developing health problems. The easiest and most common method is the body mass index (BMI). The BMI is a mathematical formula that is highly correlated with body fat, and has gained international acceptance.

Body Mass Index Table

BMI	19	20	21	22	23	24	25	26	27	28	29	30	35	40
Height (inches)	Weight in pounds													
58	91	96	100	105	110	115	119	124	129	134	138	143	167	191
59	94	99	104	109	114	119	124	128	133	138	143	148	173	198
60	97	102	107	112	118	123	128	133	138	143	148	153	179	204
61	100	106	111	116	122	127	132	137	143	148	153	158	185	211
62	104	109	115	120	126	131	136	142	147	153	158	164	191	218
63	107	113	118	124	130	135	141	146	152	158	163	169	197	225
64	110	116	122	128	134	140	145	151	157	163	169	174	204	232
65	114	120	126	132	138	144	150	156	162	168	174	180	210	240
66	118	124	130	136	142	148	155	161	167	173	179	186	216	247
67	121	127	134	140	146	153	159	166	172	178	185	191	223	255
68	125	131	138	144	151	158	164	171	177	184	190	197	230	262
69	128	135	142	149	155	162	169	176	182	189	196	203	236	270
70	132	139	146	153	160	167	174	181	188	195	202	207	243	278
71	136	143	150	157	165	172	179	186	193	200	208	215	250	286
72	140	147	154	162	169	177	184	191	199	206	213	221	258	294
73	144	151	159	166	174	182	189	197	204	212	219	227	265	302
74	148	155	163	171	179	186	194	202	210	218	225	233	272	311
75	152	160	168	176	184	192	200	208	216	224	232	240	279	319
76	156	164	172	180	189	197	205	213	221	230	238	246	287	328

If your BMI falls between 18.5 and 24.9, your weight is likely within normal range. If your BMI is under 18.5, you may be underweight and if it is over 25, you are probably overweight. A BMI over 30 is considered obese. A drawback of the BMI is that it neither distinguishes fat from muscle, nor takes into account the higher body fat content normally found in females. Using this method, a body builder could appear to be obese because of a greater muscle mass (muscle weighs more than fat).

Another method of checking your health risk is the waist-to-hip ratio, which reflects the proportion of body fat located around the abdomen. Evidence shows that an apple-shaped body (large abdomen or pot belly) is more often linked to health problems, such as heart disease and cancer, than a pear-shaped body, and is probably a bigger risk factor than a high BMI. To determine your waist-to-hip ratio, measure your waist and then your hip at the widest points and divide the first number by the second. Having a waist-to-hip ratio greater than 0.95 for men and 0.80 for women is associated with increased health risks.

The last, and perhaps most revealing, determinant of health risk is your body composition (fat vs. muscle). The preferred method is to check your percentage of body fat, which can be done using fat calipers, a bioelectric impedance device, near infrared technology or DEXA (dual energy x-ray absorptiometry). DEXA is considered the most accurate method. For women, the target body fat ranges from 15 to 25 percent, and for men, ten to 20 percent. Individuals with body fat of five percent or more above the high end of the range for their gender are considered to be obese.

Causes of Obesity

In the past, the first law of thermodynamics was often used to explain the control of body weight. Simply put, if energy intake (food) exceeds energy expenditures (exercise/

activity), then weight gain occurs. Conversely, reducing intake and increasing expenditures was believed to be the key to weight loss. For years, doctors and researchers believed this simple theory to be the answer. We now know, however, that other factors are involved. Some people can exercise religiously, reduce food intake and still not lose weight. And, of course, we all know people who can eat whatever they want and never gain a pound.

Weight gain and obesity are complex conditions, dependent upon various lifestyle, hormonal, biochemical, metabolic and genetic factors. For instance, your basal metabolic rate (BMR), the rate at which your body burns calories at rest, will have an impact on your weight and, subsequently, on your ability to lose weight. This rate is dependent on several factors, including your activity level and your thyroid gland. If your thyroid is sluggish and not functioning optimally, it can slow your metabolic rate and cause weight gain. How much, and what types of, food you consume will also play important roles. Overeating and consuming more calories than your body uses for energy can result in weight gain, regardless of whether those calories come from fat, carbohydrates or protein. Food quality also matters — eating too much saturated fat, sugar, processed food and fast food can cause hormonal changes that lead to weight gain.

Aside from food, there are numerous external and internal factors that contribute to weight gain.

Stress — Ever notice how you seem to put on weight when you are under the most pressure and least equipped to deal with it? Your workplace is in the process of major lay offs, your credit card bills are mounting and you face each day ravenously hungry — adding weight gain to your list of worries. Exposure to chronic stress can cause weight gain, particularly around the mid-section, where it is most hazardous. This occurs because stress increases the production and release of cortisol, a hormone that increases body fat storage and stimulates the appetite. Eating in response to stress can also be a learned habit, a coping mechanism that is easy to do and comforting. Many individuals turn to sweets and carbohydrates to sooth their worries, not realizing that these foods can actually worsen their emotional well-being, causing mood swings, irritability and food cravings. In either case, you need to interrupt the cycle and improve your response to stress.

Genetics — Genetics may be responsible for some cases of obesity, but experts agree that having a genetic predisposition towards obesity does not mean that this is your fate. We may take on poor dietary habits and a sedentary lifestyle as a result of the way we were raised by our parents. These attributes are not caused by flawed genes, but rather learned behaviors. Studies have shown that lifestyle factors are a much more significant determinant of weight than genetics. Your activity level, for example, is a major player in weight balance. Inactivity causes loss of muscle mass, a reduced metabolic rate and increased body fat. Conversely, regular exercise can improve muscle mass and boost metabolism. As we exercise, our muscles utilize calories for energy and generate heat, which promotes the burning of fat.

Hormones — When you think of hormonal changes, most of us think of milestones like puberty and menopause. But hormone levels can fluctuate at any age, and have a significant impact on weight. High estrogen levels, for example, are associated with weight gain. Yet, many women find that they gain weight during menopause while their estrogen levels are lower. This is because, as estrogen levels decline, the fat cells take over the production of estrogen, in order to meet the growing demand, and consequently increase in size and number. Testosterone also affects weight. Testosterone helps the body maintain lean muscle mass and burn fat. A deficiency in this hormone, as commonly occurs in women around menopause and in men over 50 years of age, can cause the loss of muscle mass, which leads to a reduced metabolism and fat gain.

Other hormones, including human growth hormone (HGH) and insulin, help regulate body weight. HGH increases lean muscle mass and reduces body fat storage. Levels decline with age, particularly after age 50, causing an increase in body fat and a decrease in muscle mass. Insulin, on the other hand, encourages fat storage. Each time we eat, food is broken down into glucose (sugar), and insulin is released to help bring glucose into the cells to be used for energy. Chronic and over-consumption of sugars and refined starches can cause higher levels of insulin, leading to insulin resistance — a precursor to Type II diabetes. As well, when insulin levels are high, the body stores more fat and is prevented from using fat as a source of energy.

Brain — The brain has a significant impact on our overall health and our body weight is no exception. Serotonin is a chemical messenger in the brain that regulates our mood, cravings and satiety. When levels are low, we feel hungry and when they are high, we feel satisfied. This is why people with depression, or women in their menstrual cycle, crave carbohydrates. Carbohydrates provide tryptophan, a necessary element that the brain uses to make serotonin. Certain weight-loss products work by elevating serotonin to promote satiety and reduce cravings for food. Satiety is also regulated by leptin, a hormone produced by body fat. Researchers have found that some people become resistant to their own leptin. To compensate for this, the body produces more and more of the hormone, but the 'satisfied' message is not property received by the brain.

Sleep — One of the most recently recognized factors that can affect body weight is lack of sleep. Sleep is vital for health and well-being, yet it is often taken for granted and the first thing to go when you have a busy schedule. Researchers have found that those who get five hours of sleep or fewer per night produce higher amounts of a hormone called ghrelin, which stimulates appetite. It can also reduce the production of HGH, the hormone that is important for regulating metabolism. As a result, lack of sleep may fuel your hunger, reduce your metabolism and contribute to the expansion of your waistline. There are many factors that affect our sleep, most importantly stress.

LIFELONG WEIGHT-MANAGEMENT STRATEGIES

Our day-to-day choices have a greater impact on our weight and overall health than any other single factor — things like packing your lunch, taking the stairs instead of the elevator, choosing low-fat frozen yogurt over ice cream. The cumulative effect of these small changes can add up to significant reductions in daily caloric intake, as well as considerable increases in the amount of energy you expend. The most effective way to achieve long-term weight loss is a five-pronged approach that includes stress management, adequate sleep, a balanced diet, consistent exercise and safe supplementation. Note: before embarking on any weight-loss program, go to your doctor for a physical exam.

Top Ten Dietary Weight-Loss Tips

Experts agree that healthy eating, rather than restrictive dieting, is the best way to lose weight and keep it off. Here are my top ten nutritional tips for achieving a healthy body weight:

1. **Eat at least three meals a day**. Or more; preferably four to five small meals to keep your metabolism and energy level optimized. Some people skip breakfast or lunch, thinking they are saving calories. Don't. Skipping meals can raise your appetite, deplete your energy levels and lead to binge eating. When you are hungry between meals, snack on healthful foods, such as fruit, yogurt, raw vegetables, nuts and seeds.

2. **Emphasize fresh unprocessed foods.** Low-fat, nutrient-dense foods — fresh fruits, vegetables, legumes (beans, peas and lentils) and whole grains — provide the most nutritional impact. But be sure to eat an assortment. We have a tendency to eat the same foods over and over, and therefore tend to get the same nutrients all the time. Eating a variety of wholesome foods is the best way to ensure you get the optimum amount of vitamins, minerals and phytochemicals you need to support lifelong health.

At the same time, cut down on processed and refined foods, as they tend to be high in calories and low in nutritional value. That means avoiding fast food, junk food, white bread, rice and pasta, candy, cookies and sweets. If you can't live without the occasional Big Mac, indulging once a week or less is probably not going to do you irreparable harm. However, if fast food is a staple of your diet, and fresh, unprocessed foods the exception, then it is time to reverse this unhealthy habit.

3. **Incorporate more fat-fighting foods into your diet.** Certain foods can actually fight fat. Soy foods, such as tofu, soy milk and tempeh, can improve fat metabolism and reduce fat absorption. Adding a scoop of flaxseed to your yogurt increases your consumption of dietary fibre and provides a rich source of lignans, which may help control hormone-related weight gain. And a cup of green tea after dinner, instead of coffee, can boost your metabolism and help you digest your meal.

4. **Limit your intake of saturated and hydrogenated fats.** Although more calorie-dense (fats provide nine calories per gram compared to only four calories per gram found in protein and carbohydrates), they fill you up more slowly than other foods because fats take longer to metabolize and absorb from the gastrointestinal tract. This causes you to eat more. And, because less chewing is required, fatty foods are consumed more quickly.

Be aware that many of the new fat-free products on the market use sugar to replace fat, providing just as many calories as the original product. For example, a cup of non-fat vanilla yogurt has 223 calories, while the whole-milk version has only 24 calories more. By the same token, using two tablespoons of jelly on a bagel instead of a tablespoon of butter gets rid of the fat but does not reduce the number of calories because of the sugar content.

It is also important to recognize that some fats, namely essential fatty acids, are 'good' fats and should not be cut out of the diet. Found in fish, nuts, seeds and vegetables, essential fatty acids are vital for health, playing important roles in the proper functioning of the brain, heart and each cell in our body.

5. **Eat an adequate amount of protein.** Protein is essential for building and maintaining lean muscle mass and requires more energy to digest, causing you to feel full longer. Without adequate protein intake, dieting and exercise can cause the body to burn muscle for fuel, lowering your basal metabolic rate — the rate at which you burn calories. The recommended amount of protein is based on body weight and activity level. For the average person, this works out to 0.4 to 0.5 grams per pound of body weight. A person who weighs 140 pounds, for example, should eat about 56 to 70 grams of protein a day. For best results, focus on eating lean protein — poultry, fish, eggs, nuts and seeds. Red meat is okay in moderation, as long as you trim the fat and watch your portion sizes. If you can't get enough protein in your diet, consider a supplement.

6. **Fill up on fibre.** Dietary fibre is a powerful asset to anyone trying to lose body fat. Dietary fibre helps balance blood sugar and insulin levels, and improves digestion and elimination. Fibre also makes us feel more full between meals because it slows digestion. Unfortunately, most North Americans only consume about ten

to 15 grams of fibre daily — less than half the amount recommended by health authorities. Ideally, you need 25 to 35 grams of fibre a day. Plant foods, such as vegetables, fruit, whole grains and legumes are excellent sources of natural fibre. Fibre is also available in supplemental form, such as powder and tablets. Read your labels carefully to ensure that you are getting a good quality product that delivers at least five to ten grams of fibre per serving.

When increasing your fibre intake, do so gradually and be sure to drink plenty of water (eight to ten glasses each day). You may notice some temporary gas or bloating as you boost your fibre intake; this is common and will subside over time.

7. **Drink at least eight glasses of water a day.** While you are losing weight, toxins stored in the fat tissue are released into your bloodstream and broken down by the liver and kidneys. Drinking plenty of pure water (up to ten, eight-ounce glasses daily) helps flush these toxins, protects against the sagging skin that may otherwise occur during fat loss and works with fibre to keep your bowels regular. Having a glass before and during meals can also help fill you up and reduce the quantity of food consumed. Heavy people need more water than thin people because they have a larger metabolic burden.

8. **Drink alcohol in moderation.** Alcohol floods the body with empty calories, providing anywhere from 20 to 120 calories per ounce. If you are going to drink, choose red wine or light beer and avoid sugary mixed drinks.

9. **Cut down on salt and sodium.** Most of the sodium in the North American diet comes from the salt shaker

and processed foods. A high-sodium diet is unhealthy and causes fluid retention, meaning it can contribute to water weight gain. If you wake up with puffiness around the eyes or swollen fingers, chances are you consume too much sodium.

10. **Consider taking a well-balanced multivitamin/mineral supplement.** As you are reducing your calorie intake, you may also be reducing your nutrient intake. A high-quality multivitamin can help fill any dietary gaps. Nutritional deficiencies are not only hard on your health, they are also hard on your weight-loss program because they can cause food cravings and binge eating.

Physical Activity for Weight Loss

Lack of physical activity is a major factor in our obesity epidemic. Modern life offers fewer opportunities for burning calories. We tend to live farther from work, necessitating long commutes. Many neighbourhoods lack sidewalks for safe walking. Even our leisure activities have become increasingly sedentary — the television and computer have replaced walking and cycling. According to a recent survey, only 34 percent of obese individuals participate in moderate physical activity. Clearly, a lack of exercise is fueling this epidemic.

The fact is, exercise can be fun and pays sizeable dividends in your weight-loss program! You can certainly reduce your weight by reducing your calorie intake. But by adding a 30-minute brisk walk four days a week, you can double your rate of weight loss. Boost that to five days a week and you can lose three times as much fat as those who exercise only two or three times a week.

With today's busy lifestyles, you may think that you don't

have the time or can't afford to exercise. The truth is there are many ways that we can incorporate moderate physical activity into our daily lifestyle — doing moderate house-work, gardening, washing the car, dancing, brisk walking. And the time need not be constraining. Although the guidelines released by the National Academies Institute of Medicine recommend that adults should spend at least one hour each day in moderately intense physical activity, regardless of weight, you can always split that into half-hour or even 15-minute intervals. Every little bit helps.

To maximize fat loss, you need to consider a regular exercise program that includes a combination of aerobic (cardiovascular) activity, toning/strengthening training and stretching. (See Chapter Three: Fitness)

Supplements for Weight Loss

Healthy eating and exercise are the foundation of a successful, long-lasting fat-loss program. However, certain nutritional supplements, when used properly, can be helpful in supporting your program. Below are my top recommended supplements to aid fat loss.

Conjugated Linoleic Acid — Conjugated linoleic acid (CLA) is a naturally occurring fatty acid found most abundantly in beef and dairy fats. Several clinical studies have found CLA supplements to be effective in promoting weight loss, without unpleasant side effects. Specifically, CLA acts to stimulate the breakdown of stored fat in the fat cells, reduce the number of existing fat cells and prevent fat stor-age, thereby helping to reduce body fat while maintaining or increasing lean muscle mass. The recommended dosage is four grams (four capsules) daily.

Green Tea — Green tea can facilitate weight loss by increasing thermogenesis, the rate at which the body burns calories. This effect is due to an interaction between its high content of potent antioxidants, and caffeine. These antioxidants are called polyphenols, specifically the catechin epigallocatechin gallate (EGCG). In one study, participants given a standardized extract, providing 375 mg green tea catechins per capsule daily, lost an average of 4.5 percent body fat. Most studies documenting the health benefits of green tea have involved three to ten cups per day. Since most people are unlikely to consume that much tea, tablets and capsules may be more convenient. Look for a product that is standardized for total polyphenol content and/or catechin concentrations. Most products provide 60 to 97 percent polyphenols and/or EGCG.

Hydroxycitric Acid — Hydroxycitric acid (HCA) is a compound derived from the fruit *Garcinia cambogia*, which is native to South and Southeast Asia. HCA supports weight loss by reducing appetite, enhancing the breakdown of fat and inhibiting fat storage, without affecting the central nervous system. There may be other benefits, and newer research has found that it can reduce cholesterol and triglycerides. While earlier studies found benefits in dosages around 1,200 to 1,500 mg HCA daily, newer research supports greater benefits at a higher dosage, such as 2,800 mg per day. No serious side effects have been reported with HCA.

Phase 2® Standardized White Kidney Bean Extract — Phase 2® is an extract of the white kidney bean that promotes weight loss by temporarily neutralizing starches from the diet. It works by inhibiting the action of an enzyme called alpha-amylase, the enzyme responsible for breaking down starches into sugar. Because less starch is digested and absorbed, calorie intake is reduced, after-meal blood sugar levels are lowered and the body is encouraged to burn stored fat.

In several clinical studies, Phase 2® has been shown to reduce the amount of sugar absorbed from starchy meals and to promote fat loss. A study conducted at the Northridge Hospital Medical Center, UCLA found those given Phase 2® lost an average of four pounds of body fat after eight weeks, experienced an average 26-point drop in triglycerides, and had more energy. In another study of 60 overweight individuals, the average weight loss was 6.45 pounds over 30 days. The recommended dosage is 1,000 to 1,500 mg before starchy meals. Phase 2® is very safe and well-tolerated, and not known to interact with any drugs or supplements.

Proteinase Inhibitor II — A protein extract derived from potatoes, Proteinase Inhibitor II works in the intestine to signal the release of a naturally occurring compound called cholecystokinin (CCK), one of the key hormones involved in hunger control. Normally released in the blood after a meal, CCK acts on the stomach to slow emptying, making you feel full, and triggers feelings of satiety (satisfaction) in the brain, thus reducing food intake. Unlike other appetite suppressants, Proteinase Inhibitor II does not contain any stimulants, so it won't affect blood pressure or heart rate.

GETTING STARTED

It is one thing to know what it takes to lose weight and keep it off. It is another thing to implement it. Having a clear-cut strategy can make the transition easier, and help you stick to your plan. Try to focus on the process rather then the end result and the pounds will come off on their own.

Keep a Food Diary

Before you decide what you need to change, take an objective look at what you are eating now. Most people underestimate the number of calories they eat by about 20 percent. To get a true idea of your current calorie consumption, keep a food diary for a week or two, being sure to record everything you eat in a day. Once you get an accurate look at what you are really eating, keep the nutrient-rich foods in your diet and whittle down the fillers — refined carbohydrates, sweets, snack foods.

Set Manageable Goals

A 50-pound weight loss is daunting. Focus on five-pound increments instead. If you gradually lose one-half to one pound a week, you will lose five pounds in five to ten weeks, while shaking off some of your fattening habits and adopting healthier ones. Reinforce your good habits by rewarding yourself as you reach each new milestone.

Make Health-Promoting Changes Daily

Everyday offers an opportunity to make healthier choices. If you like to snack, choose fresh fruit over a candy bar. Opt for low-fat sunflower seeds over high-fat potato chips.

Order your mocha without whipped cream. Look for ways to increase your exercise as well. Park your car farther away from your destination, so you do a little more walking. Wash your car by hand instead of going through the car wash. All of these small shifts in behaviour add up to steady weight loss and improved overall health.

Take Pride in Your Progress

Modest losses can yield impressive health benefits. By losing ten pounds, you can lower your blood pressure significantly. When you lose 20 excess pounds you reduce your risk of mortality by 20 to 25 percent, lessen angina symptoms by 91 percent and cut your risk of developing diabetes by more than 50 percent!

Don't Rely on Your Scale to Measure Success

The bathroom scale only tells you how much you weigh. It does not tell you what your body composition is, or whether you are carrying excess fat. In fact, if you are exercising, losing body fat and gaining lean muscle mass, it is possible that you may notice either no change in the scale or even a slight increase in weight initially. Instead, measure your success by looking in the mirror for changes in your shape, judging how your clothes fit and monitoring your body fat.

Appearance — Skin

By Dr. Paul Cohen, BA, MD, FRCPC, DABD

Dermatologist

Nicole, a publicist with a high-profile PR firm, always had healthy skin. Even as a teenager, people commented on her flawless complexion. But, over time, years of sun tanning and smoking had taken their toll, making her appear much older than her 42 years. Lines had developed around her eyes, her brow and her mouth. Her once porcelain-like complexion had become ruddy in texture and prone to redness and flushing. Worst of all, she began to get acne for the first time in her life. Embarrassed by her appearance, she hid behind hats and large sun glasses. Usually an outgoing person, she was increasingly reserved, preferring to stay out of the spotlight. Her work and social life had begun to suffer.

Some people seem immune to the effects of aging. Their skin gives off a radiant and youthful glow even as they enter mid-life and beyond. Other people, like Nicole, look old before their time. Premature aging saps their skin of vitality, leaving it dull, rough and heavily lined. Thankfully, how well or how poorly your skin ages is largely within your power. And the sooner you take control, the better the prognosis.

We all enter the world with a virtually flawless complexion, and with each day our skin suffers environmental and internal insults. Ultimately, how well you age depends on how well you protect your skin from these insults, and how well equipped you are to cope with them. From a genetic perspective, some people and skin types simply have more resources to stave off the effects of premature aging. If your parents have skin that is resistant to wrinkling, chances are you will too. More important however is the way you care for your skin. Damage to the skin can take years, even decades, to show up. Like Nicole, you may not see the ill effects of a lifetime of outdoor sports, or summers spent soaking up rays on the beach slathered in baby oil, until you enter middle age.

By that time, the damage can be psychological as well as cosmetic. Skin has a tremendous impact on how we look and feel. In a culture that reveres youth, healthy vital skin is a prized possession. When we begin to feel it slipping away, we can experience self-consciousness, embarrassment, even lower self-esteem. And the phenomenon no longer applies exclusively to women. Men too are increasingly using skin products and treatments in the hopes of keeping the effects of aging at bay. Combined, we spend an estimated US$38.3 billion globally a year on skin-care products!

The fact is beautiful skin doesn't come in a bottle. Although your skin may appreciate the care and attention you give it from the outside, no amount of creams, cosmetic procedures or beauty treatments will make up for the damage done if you smoke, drink too much alcohol and do not eat properly or get enough sleep. Beautiful skin on the outside begins with good health on the inside, and is maintained by vigilant preventative care.

UNDERSTANDING SKIN

As the body's largest organ, the skin plays a number of roles in our health. It protects the body from outside insults and infection. It regulates temperature through sweat. And it conveys our sense of touch. As we age, all of these functions become impaired, and so does the cosmetic appearance of our skin.

Skin Structure

The skin is composed of three basic layers: the epidermis, the dermis and a fat layer. Each of these layers will have an impact on how well your skin ages.

The epidermis — The epidermis is the skin's outer layer and is home to a number of important cells. On the very outer surface of the epidermis is the stratum corneum, a protective coating of dead skin cells that forms when fresh cells, made in the skin's deeper layers, push their way to the surface, flatten and die. This layer is thinner than a sheet of tissue paper, and functions to help hold in moisture and oil.

The stratum corneum is continually sloughed off as new cells take its place. As we age, this process slows down. In a young person, cell turnover occurs about every 28 to 30 days. By the time we're in our 60s, the process takes 45 to

50 days, which is one of the reasons our skin loses the freshness of youth.

At the bottom of the epidermis are the basal cells, which produce new skin cells. The epidermis also contains melanocytes; cells that produce melanin. The actual tone and colour of your skin depends on its unique amount and concentration of melanin. By the late 30s to early 40s, the melanocytes begin to burn out, reducing the skin's ability to fight sun damage and causing pigmentation to become uneven.

The dermis — Under the epidermis is the dermis, which makes up 90 percent of the thickness of your skin. The dermis is the skin's nerve centre. It contains nerve receptors — which are sensitive to pressure, temperature and pain — and sebaceous and sweat glands — which produce skin protective oil — as well as hair follicles and blood vessels.

Sweat and sebaceous glands help produce the skin's acid mantle, a thin coating of oil and perspiration that helps protect from bacterial and fungal infections. Often we unwittingly strip the acid mantle away through use of harsh soaps, and disrupt the skin's natural pH balance. After age 30, the oil glands reduce their production significantly and the loss continues over the years. The sweat glands also slowly lose their ability to function, making it harder for your body to regulate itself and register heat and cold.

The dermis also contains a dense meshwork of collagen and elastin, two types of protein that give your skin its strength and elasticity. In youth, the skin's supply of collagen and elastin is constantly replenished by fibroblasts. As we age, the dermis thins and the fibroblasts lose their ability to function. Less and less collagen and elastin are produced, and the skin begins to lose firmness. At the same time, the nerves, cells and mechanisms that repair sun damage — and register the presence of foreign agents and toxins — can become exhausted. Free-radical damage becomes more pronounced, accelerating aging.

The fat layer — Under the dermis, the fat layer serves to insulate and protect your inner organs, and acts as a cushion that helps keep the skin plump and smooth. At about age 40, and increasingly thereafter, the fat layer thins, causing the skin to lose its plump youthful softness and become more fragile and likely to abrade.

Skin Tone

Your skin tone and type will play a significant role in determining the impact of age on your outward appearance. White skin scars and discolours less easily, so acne scars are often less noticeable, while brown skin is more immune to fine lines but vulnerable to scarring and discolouration, even from minor acne.

White skin — White skin is more susceptible to skin damage, ruddiness and photo aging from repeated exposure to sunlight. It is also prone to broken blood vessels and capillaries, especially along the cheeks and sides of the nose. Melanin, the compound that determines skin colour, absorbs the sun's rays. People with little or no melanin have few natural defences. Very pale people, who took in a great deal of sun in their youth and had multiple sun burns, can age prematurely and severely.

White skin is also more prone to rosacea, a condition

characterized by flushing, blushing and redness to the face, as well as pre-cancerous and cancerous skin lesions. The fairer the skin, the more vulnerable it is. On the upside, it is more forgiving. White skin scars and discolours less easily, whether from injury or acne, so it generally responds well to cosmetic procedures like dermabrasion, deep acid peels and cosmetic surgery.

Brown skin — Brown skin contains more melanin and a greater density of sebaceous or oil glands than white skin. As a result it is less likely to sustain sun damage, to develop skin cancer or to have freckles or sun spots, and more likely to remain smooth and wrinkle-free longer.

For the same reason, it is also more vulnerable to damage from acne and injuries. Because of its high melanin content, brown skin is extremely susceptible to inflammation. A mild case of acne can trigger an extreme inflammatory reaction, and elicit the production of chemicals that swiftly attack and break down the elastin in skin. This can lead to visible scarring, changes in pigment and large raised scars called keloids. It is also why a minor scratch or pimple can leave a dark spot, called post-inflammatory hyper pigmentation. Many state-of-the-art procedures cause some initial injury or inflammation to the skin, and can result in scarring in pigmented skin, limiting the number of procedures available for brown skin.

Light brown/yellow skin — Extra melanin gives Mediterranean and Asian skin many of the good and many of the problematic qualities of brown skin. Asian skin is more resistant to sun damage than white skin, and unlike brown skin tends to have very tiny pores, giving the skin a very smooth appearance. Mediterranean skin tends to be thicker and oilier, making it less susceptible to sun damage and wrinkles. Both types are vulnerable to discolouration and extreme inflammatory responses. A simple pimple can leave a lasting mark.

Gender Differences

With the exception of acne, which is more common with age in women than men, the prevalence of most skin disorders is probably equally divided between the sexes. There are however notable differences between male and female skin. Men tend to have thicker skin than women because of testosterone, the dominant male hormone, and therefore have more natural barriers to aging and trauma. They often have more sweat and oil glands as well. With regular shaving, the skin on the lower face is exfoliated but on the upper face the oil glands can get very thick. Shaving also makes skin on the lower face more sensitive to irritation, particularly for brown-skinned men, who are vulnerable to ingrown hairs, persistent folliculitis and razor burn.

Women, on the other hand, tend to have thinner skin and to produce less oil than men, particularly as they grow older. Not only does this make them more likely to experience dry skin, but their skin also becomes a less efficient barrier against irritants, allergens and bacteria, and is more susceptible to dermatitis, trauma and infections. With age, the hormone levels begin to drop and the skin becomes more fragile for both sexes. In women, the drop in hormone activity is more dramatic and has a greater effect.

SKIN PROBLEMS

In your 40s and 50s you probably think aging of the skin is going to be your biggest concern. And to some degree that is true. Your skin will start to lose the blush of youth. Fine lines may develop into deeper lines, particularly between the eyebrows. Skin may become coarse in texture, dull and less elastic. Uneven pigmentation, freckles and broken blood vessels are often more apparent. And problems of large pores, dark circles and liver spots become more pronounced. Some people will notice thinning of the hair and brittleness of the nails as well.

What you may be surprised to learn is that problems you thought were restricted to adolescence often come full circle in mid-life. It is not unusual to experience acne for the first time in your 40s, particularly in women. For fair skinned people, rosacea commonly becomes a problem at this time. The risk of certain health conditions, such as skin cancer, also increases dramatically after middle age.

There are a number of reasons for these changes. First and foremost is the sun. The sun damage you had in the beginning of your life will start to wreak havoc on your skin around your 40s or 50s, just as the repair process starts to slow. Hormone changes will contribute as well. As estrogen levels drop with menopause, so will the skin's ability to maintain moisture and elasticity. In some cases the changes may be exacerbated by cessation of birth control hormone therapy. Once you go off the pill, you can start to break out.

Sun Damage

Time is not your skin's greatest enemy; the environment is. A certain amount of wrinkling will develop as a result of aging, genetics and repetitive movements made over a life-time, but the way you care for your skin and the toxins it is exposed to will have a much greater impact. The biggest threats to your skin's health are:

- Sun exposure
- Cigarette smoke
- Environmental toxins
- Poor diet
- Excess alcohol
- Stress
- Harsh soaps or detergent-based moisturizers
- Sleep deprivation

The vast majority of wrinkles are caused by sun damage. Sun rays are classified as UVB or UVA. UVB, the 'tanning ray', is strongest in the summer months and is responsible for tanning and burning the epidermis of the skin. This manifests in very obvious signs of inflammation — redness, irritation, warmth — all of which damage and age the skin. Contrary to popular belief, there is no such thing as a safe or 'base' tan. Tanned skin provides an SPF of two. While you may not burn, you are getting a tremendous amount of UV damage.

What you don't see is what you should be most worried about. UVA rays were once touted as the 'safe ray' because they do not cause the skin to burn, but we have since learned that they actually do the most amount of damage to the skin, causing subclinical inflammation. And, because UVA rays are the same strength year round and are able to penetrate window glass, they inflict continuous insults on the skin. In fact, most wrinkling and fine lines are caused by day-to-day sun exposure to UVA. Unfortunately, many people do not wear sunscreen everyday because the signs of UVA damage are not immediately obvious.

Acne

Acne becomes an unfortunate reality for some adults as they enter middle age, and psychologically is much more devastating to a 40-year-old than a 14-year-old. It is not yet known exactly what causes adult acne, but dermatologists have linked it to hormone fluctuations and to rich anti-aging creams and moisturizers, which may explain why the condition is so much more common in women than men.

Breakouts most commonly appear on the face, back and chest — areas where there is a concentration of sebaceous and oil glands. For people prone to acne, wrinkle treatments can wreak havoc on the skin, blocking pores and exacerbating the condition. The exception is found in retinoic acid-derivative creams, which can treat wrinkles and acne. Although acne cannot be cured, it can be controlled with oil-free, non-comedogenic cleansers and acne treatments (non-comedogenic products do not clog the pores and will not cause acne). It may take some experimenting to find what works for your skin. Sixty percent of adult women with acne either do not respond to standard acne treatments or build up a tolerance to frequently prescribed medications such as antibiotics.

Rosacea

An estimated 14 million North Americans suffer from rosacea, but most sufferers fail to realize they have the condition. A Gallup survey found that 78 percent of the public has no knowledge of rosacea, including how to recognize it and what to do about it. Often the early signs of rosacea are mistaken for something else, such as sunburn, acne or even alcoholism.

Rosacea is a chronic disorder that primarily affects the cheeks, chin, nose or central forehead, and is often characterized by flare-ups and remissions. It typically first appears after age 30 as a flushing or redness that comes and goes. Over time, the redness becomes ruddier and more persistent and visible blood vessels may appear. Bumps and pimples often develop, and in some people the eyes feel irritated and appear bloodshot. In other cases, the nose may become swollen and enlarged from excess tissue. Without treatment, each of these potential signs and symptoms may progress from mild to moderate to severe.

Unfortunately, if you are prone to rosacea there is not much you can do to prevent it. It can, however, be effectively controlled with medical therapy, anti-redness creams containing vitamin C, herbal extracts or niacinimide and lifestyle changes, such as avoiding spicy food, hot beverages and red wine. Because sun damage may bring rosacea on more quickly, it is important that susceptible people use sunscreen with a high SPF, preferably in a non-comedogenic lotion.

Skin Cancer

Skin cancer can affect a person at any age, but the effects of sun damage in early life often begin to take their toll in the 40s and 50s. People who have a history of taking in a lot of sun, who spend a great deal of time outdoors, who are fair skinned, have multiple moles or who have a family history of cancer are at particular risk. There are three different types of skin cancer: basal cell, squamous cell and melanoma. Fortunately skin cancer is very preventable and, when caught early, is a very treatable disease.

Basal cell skin cancer — Basal cell skin cancer is the most common form of skin cancer and will affect one in seven Canadians. Basal cell skin cancer appears as a pearly bump or mole that is new, doesn't heal or persistently bleeds. These occur most commonly on sun exposed areas — the face, head and neck, and on the back, chest and the back of the legs. Fortunately, basal cell skin cancer is very treatable. The cancerous area is simply excised. But, if left to develop, it can be cosmetically disfiguring, particularly on areas like the face and hands. People prone to basal cell bumps need to protect their skin from the sun very carefully, and have their skin examined regularly.

Squamous cell cancer — Potentially more serious is squamous cell carcinoma. Characterized by pink/reddish bumps on the skin that tend to bleed and grow, but do not heal, squamous cell carcinoma occurs most commonly on sun-exposed skin, such as the head, face and neck. Depending on where they occur, this cancer can be quite serious. Squamous cell cancer bumps found on the lips and ears, two areas people often forget to protect with sunscreen, are more likely to spread to other parts of the body.

Melanoma — Melanoma, the least common but most serious form of skin cancer, kills approximately 800 Canadians every year, and is expected to claim more lives over the next 20 years as the baby boomers enter old age. This type of cancer manifests as a mole that changes size, shape or colour, and most commonly appears on the back, an area that is difficult to monitor. If caught early, melanoma can be treated with surgical excision of the mole.

CARING FOR YOUR SKIN

Your best protection against premature aging is sunscreen. Redness, broken blood vessels and pre-cancerous changes can take ten to 20 years to develop. Prevention simply cannot be over emphasized, and it is never too late to adopt good habits. Even in your 40s you can make a significant difference to how your skin will look 20 years down the road.

A broad spectrum sunscreen that protects against both UVA and UVB rays, and has an SPF of at least 15, should be a part of every person's daily skin-care regime. It takes about 30 ml of sunscreen to cover the entire body, so apply thickly for full protection. If you spend more than two hours outdoors in the sun, re-apply the sunscreen every few hours; more frequently if sweating or swimming. If you are balding, don't forget your scalp.

It should be noted that sunscreen is only one piece of the puzzle; it is not a license to lie on the beach and deliberately tan. Avoid midday sun when UVB rays are at their highest, and be sure to wear hats, sun glasses and long sleeves. In the winter, apply sunscreen daily over your moisturizer. Be cognizant that make-up containing SPF only provides limited protection, and may degrade during the day, providing a much lower SPF than indicated on the package.

Lifestyle
Beautiful skin on the outside begins with good health on the inside. Getting adequate sleep, managing your stress

levels and eating a healthy diet will go a long way toward preserving your skin's health. Recent evidence suggests that certain foods may be especially restorative for skin. Essential fatty acids — namely omega-3 and omega-6 — are 'good' fats found in fish, nuts and seeds. They are shown to help repair skin, hair and nails and help control inflammation. Of these, omega-3 fatty acids are particularly important. Omega-3 fatty acids have the ability to reduce the body's production of inflammatory compounds dramatically, but to work properly must exist in balance with omega-6 fatty acids. Unfortunately the North American diet tends to be heavy on omega-6 and low on omega-3. The best sources of omega-3 fatty acids are salmon, mackerel, herring, anchovies, snapper, bass, bluefish and trout — or a daily fish oil supplement.

There is evidence that antioxidants, abundant in fruits and vegetables, also have a positive impact on skin health by fighting free-radical damage. Vitamin C, for example, is shown to stimulate collagen, giving skin a taut appearance and helping with prevention of wrinkles. It also stabilizes the blood vessels and may be beneficial in treating broken blood vessels. Alpha lipoic acid, also a powerful antioxidant, is a constituent in the extra cellular matrix of the skin, where the collagen and elastin flows, and may help maintain the skin's elasticity. Alpha hydroxy acid and beta hydroxy acid, two of the first antioxidants to be included in skin-care products, exfoliate and encourage cell turnover and renewal of skin, keeping it smooth.

Antioxidants appear to be effective whether taken orally, either through diet or a nutritional supplement, or applied topically, and are increasingly being incorporated into skin products.

Skin Products

Despite our penchant for skin-care products, skin creams cannot miraculously reverse the signs of aging. But there is evidence that certain products may help. Vitamin A acid-derivative creams, available by prescription, are scientifically proven to prevent and treat fine lines, stimulate collagen and promote turnover of upper layers of skin, making it appear smoother. Glycolic acid creams, available in over the counter products, are shown to cause exfoliation, helping to rid the skin of dullness and to reduce fine lines when used in conjunction with sunscreen, particularly if you start treatment before significant problems appear. Both types of creams can be irritating for certain skin types.

For best results pair your wrinkle treatment with a daily skin-care regime suited to your skin type:

Dry skin — A gentle skin-care routine can help make dry skin more supple and radiant. People with dry skin should cleanse with 'super-fatted' soaps that contain emollients like olive oil, shea butter or glycerin, and moisturize with creams containing humectants like urea, lactic acid and hyaluronic acid. Emollients prevent the evaporation of moisture, while humectants draw water from deep in the skin up to the surface. The drier the skin, the more hydrating the moisturizer should be.

Oily skin — With oily skin there is a temptation to over strip. Avoid it. Harsh detergent-based soaps and alcohol-laden astringents that dry up oil can damage your skin in the long run, and encourage already overactive oil glands to step up production. Instead, use oil-binding liquid or gel cleaners and do not wash more than twice a day. People with oily skin may not need moisturizer. If you choose to moisturize, use a lotion that contains humectants, such as glycerin or sodium pyrrolidonecarboxyic acid (PCA), and a gel-based or spray sunscreen. Lotions are lighter than creams and tend to contain less oil, so they won't clog pores. Newer moisturizers may have a clay base so they do not look as shiny.

Combination skin — If your T-zone is very oily, use a glycolic acid-based astringent, as opposed to one with alcohol, once a day and a light moisturizer with hyaluronic acid or lactic acid only where you need it, usually on the cheeks. The last thing you want to do is make an already oily T-zone even oilier.

Non-Invasive Cosmetic Treatments

With recent advancements, there are a number of non-invasive cosmetic procedures that produce dramatic effects on fine lines and sun damage without causing significant damage to the skin. Unfortunately, the options for darker skin are limited. Current treatments work by irritating the skin and may cause discoloration and uneven pigmentation in brown skin if used incorrectly.

Peels — Peels use natural acids like glycolic acid to exfoliate the outer layers of the skin, and are shown to prevent fine lines, stimulate cell turnover and renewal and clean out the skin. For this reason, peels are indicated for people breaking out, and for men with thick oil glands on the upper face. Although the results are not seen quickly, peels can make a significant difference over the years when used in conjunction with sunscreen, but may be irritating to sensitive skin and rosacea. Peels should be used with caution on darker skin.

Microdermabrasion — Microdermabrasion uses crystals to exfoliate the skin. In studies, microdermabrasion is shown to stimulate precursors to collagen, so it may in fact plump the skin in addition to sloughing off the top layer. Though widely offered, microdermabrasion can be irritating for sensitive skin and should only be done by a dermatologist or cosmetic surgeon, particularly on darker skin where it can cause discolouration.

Botox — The most popular treatment of the past decade, botox relaxes muscles in the face with botulinum toxin. Injected into the skin this toxin can prevent lines caused by repetitive movements, such as crows' feet or frown lines between the brows, and is safe for all skin types. Results last about four months but the earlier you start the more fine lines you can prevent.

IPL laser — Commonly referred to as photorejuvenation, the Intense Pulsed Light (IPL) laser can erase much of the damage caused by the sun, helping get rid of age spots, uneven skin tone and broken blood vessels. It can also be used to constrict blood vessels and prevent redness and flushing in people with rosacea. IPL lasers are not appropriate for dark skin, which doesn't tend to get a lot of age spots anyway, and should only be used with caution on Asian skin.

Appearance — Smile

By Dr. Steven Young, DMD, Cert Pros, FRCD(C)

Prosthodontist

Your smile is often the first thing people notice about you. And, if not up to par, is often the first thing we hide. Stained, broken or missing teeth can be as psychologically devastating as blemished skin, and may even impact your opportunities in life. A 1998 survey by the American Academy of Cosmetic Dentistry showed that people with defective teeth are more likely to experience social and employment discrimination. Half of the respondents saw unattractive teeth as a sign of poor personal hygiene.

We get one permanent set of teeth. With good care it can last a lifetime, provided we make adjustments for age. Studies indicate that older people have the highest rates of periodontal disease. At least half of people over age 55 have periodontitis, a condition that affects the structures that support the teeth. Almost one out of four people age 65 and older have lost all of their teeth. Clearly, as we age we need to do more to maintain good oral health

What you may not realize is that oral health is not just important for maintaining a nice-looking smile and being able to eat corn on the cob; it is essential to quality of life. Every tooth in your mouth plays an important role in speaking, chewing and maintaining proper alignment of other teeth. Just a few loose or missing teeth can make biting into fresh fruits and vegetables difficult, even painful, and make it more difficult to obtain adequate nutrition. What's more, recent research suggests that periodontal disease is linked to a number of major health concerns such as heart disease, stroke, respiratory disease and diabetes.

THE AGING MOUTH

As we age, our teeth are more prone to root cavities, which can be more difficult to treat than surface cavities. With age, our teeth become more susceptible to receding gums, which expose areas of the root, making it more vulnerable to decay.

We are also more likely to be taking medication, much of which can cause side effects such as dry mouth, soft tissue changes, taste changes and gingival overgrowth. Not only can these side effects be unpleasant, but they can also leave you susceptible to tooth decay and periodontal disease. Dry mouth, for instance, leaves you without enough saliva to wash away food and neutralize plaque. This in turn can cause a sore throat, problems with speaking, difficulty swallowing and hoarseness. Some common culprits are antihistamines, diuretics, pain killers, high blood pressure medications and antidepressants.

At the same time, teeth become less sensitive as we get older, so it becomes more difficult to detect potential problems. You could have a cavity or the onset of gum disease but not experience any pain or obvious symptoms.

Changes in the mouth are particularly common among menopausal or post-menopausal women. Recent studies suggest that estrogen deficiency could place post-menopausal women at higher risk for severe periodontal disease and tooth loss. In addition, hormonal changes in older women may result in discomfort in the mouth, including dry mouth, pain and burning sensations in the gum tissue and altered taste; especially salty, peppery or sour.

ORAL HEALTH AND DISEASE RISK

Recent research has linked oral health to general health. Gum disease is a risk factor for several major health concerns, including diabetes, heart disease and stroke. While the reasons for the link between mouth health and general health are not yet known, one theory cites harmful bacteria, which can build up in the spaces between teeth and gums. If disrupted, these pockets of bacteria can enter the bloodstream and settle elsewhere in the body, causing damage to other organs, such as the heart.

Heart disease — Researchers have found that people with periodontal disease are almost twice as likely to suffer from coronary artery disease as those without. A recent study discovered that the same type of bacteria found in the plaque on our teeth can also be found on the walls of the arteries. And periodontal disease can exacerbate existing heart conditions. The American Academy of Periodontology reports that patients at risk for infective endocarditis may require antibiotics prior to dental procedures.

Diabetes — Research also shows a link between gum disease and the likelihood of having diabetes. A recent University of Buffalo study shows gum disease may be more prevalent among diabetic patients than non-diabetic people. Diabetics are more likely to suffer severe bone loss, tooth loss and infections from gum disease. While one condition does not cause the other, gum disease may affect the severity of diabetes, making treatment more difficult.

Stroke — Studies have pointed to a relationship between periodontal disease and stroke. In one study that looked at the causal relationship of oral infection as a risk factor for stroke, people diagnosed with acute cerebrovascular ischemia were found more likely to have an oral infection when compared to those in the control group.

Osteoporosis — There is some evidence that a relationship between osteoporosis and periodontal disease exists. Bone loss is associated with both periodontal disease and osteoporosis. It is suspected that osteoporosis could lead to tooth loss because the density of the bone that supports the teeth may be decreased.

TEETH FOR LIFE

Good oral care starts at home. Brush your teeth and tongue at least twice a day to remove plaque and bacteria that cause gum disease, bad breath and cavities. One of these times should be before bed. Much of the plaque and germ buildup that causes gum disease and cavities occurs during the night. A good oral health routine also means flossing once a day; about one-third of tooth surface is between the teeth, where your toothbrush can't reach. Flossing also helps to counteract caries, a chemical process that affects all surfaces of the tooth when sugars are transformed into acids.

Use proper technique — Avoid a back-and-forth motion when brushing, as it may force plaque and bacteria under the gum line. Instead, brush on a 45 degree angle, using a rotation movement, or starting from the gum and moving along the tooth surface to brush plaque away from the gums. A good brushing takes two to three minutes.

Custom care — There is no one-size-fits-all dental program. Your teeth are individual to you and may need special care and attention. If you have sensitive teeth, you may need special toothpaste, or a toothbrush with extra-soft bristles, to help combat discomfort. Depending on the oral health needs of your family, individuals may need separate toothpastes, or require the services of a specialist, such as a periodontist or endodontist.

Check your mouth — Periodontal disease and tooth decay are the leading causes of tooth loss in older adults. Check your mouth regularly for symptoms of gum disease — bleeding when you brush or floss, red and shiny gums or swelling of the gums. Gum disease can be prevented and easily reversed if caught in the early stages.

Diet — Eating a well-balanced diet that is abundant in healthy foods and low in sugar helps prevent gum disease and maintain good oral health. Sugar mixes with the bacteria in your mouth and forms a mild acid that attacks the tooth's enamel and can eventually cause cavities. The frequency and duration of sugar exposure is also significant. It is more damaging to sip a sugary soft drink or suck a hard candy over a long period of time than it is to eat a sugary sweet, like pie or pastry.

Some foods can actually help teeth fight tooth decay and guard against cavities, while contributing to good overall health and wellness. Eating raw, crunchy fruit and vegetables, like celery and apples, after a meal helps stimulate saliva and wash sugar away from the teeth. Dairy products, including cheese and milk, also help prevent tooth decay by neutralizing the acid that causes caries and by diffusing plaque.

Butt out — Tobacco is a major contributor to gum disease and may also be a factor in oral cancer. Not only do tobacco products stain your teeth and cause bad breath, but they can also irritate the area under the gums, which is where gum disease begins. In addition, tobacco will cause the blood vessels in your gums to constrict, making the tissue less healthy and leaving it vulnerable to infection.

See your dentist regularly — Visit your dentist every six months to treat problems before it is too late. A periodontal evaluation is especially important if you notice any symptoms of periodontal disease, have heart disease, diabetes, respiratory disease, osteoporosis or have a sore or irritation in your mouth that does not get better within two weeks. If a member of your family has periodontal disease, you are at increased risk. Research suggests the bacteria that cause periodontal disease can pass through saliva. This means the common contact of saliva puts children and couples at risk for contracting periodontal disease through another family member.

Stress

By Dr. Richard Earle, PhD
Canadian Institute of Stress

George, a small-town minister of 19 years, was 50 pounds overweight and suffering from ulcers at age 46. Five or six times a year he was immobilized by lower back pain. Torn between the demands of home and congregation, all he could think about was making it to the end of the week. George realized he was not only shortchanging his congregation but also his family and himself, and had to learn to budget his time better.

Marion, an architect by training, was noticeably underweight and appeared much older than her years. Her face was deeply lined, with dark circles under her eyes, and her voice was husky, like that of a person who had been up all night. At 35 years of age she looked like someone in her early to mid-50s.

Bill, age 42, was an executive on the fast track. Admired for his physical and mental energy, he was

> *always brimming with fresh ideas and the ability to see*
> *them through. For as long as anyone could remember,*
> *he'd been a fierce competitor in sports, as well as the*
> *life of any party he attended. But, unknown to most*
> *of his friends, Bill had regular spells of extreme and*
> *crippling fatigue. By the time he finally went to see*
> *his doctor, exhaustion was threatening to take over his*
> *life.*

Like George, Marion and Bill, most of us have noticed changes in our bodies and energy levels as we have grown older. We may play a hard game of tennis and discover we are stiff for days. Or we may go out with friends, have a few too many drinks and wake up the next morning with a hangover that seems way out of proportion with our indiscretion.

Studies have shown that as many as 20 percent of adults in Canada and the United States feel many years older than their chronological age would suggest. We call this condition premature aging. Although anyone, from teenagers to the elderly, may experience it, adults between 40 and 50 are by far the most vulnerable.

The culprit: stress. Not simply stress in and of itself, but stress that becomes larger than life, wreaking havoc on the body's systems. And when stress runs out of control in this way, it can speed up the aging process, sapping vitality, weakening the immune system and causing a host of troubling symptoms.

Unfortunately, the symptoms of accelerated aging are so much a part of many people's lives that they are often taken for granted. If you're easily fatigued, if your body aches, if you frequently feel tense, if you find yourself dragging through the day at work and then collapsing the moment you walk through the door, you're probably in danger. Or perhaps you simply don't feel like yourself — the self who once approached life with boundless energy and a store-house of enthusiasm.

In 1980, researchers at the Canadian Institute of Stress undertook a 15-year investigation into the effects of stress on the human body. Each of the 3,138 participants who completed the study underwent rigorous testing for signs of stress-related aging, and followed an individually tailored plan to restore depleted vitality.

Every one of the 1,692 women and 1,577 men who started the study tested older than their calendar ages, many by ten years or more. But at the end of eight months, the group had reduced body age by an average of 11 years. Overall, blood pressure was down. Muscles became more flexible. Posture grew more erect. Vision and skin tone improved; wrinkles became far less noticeable.

While these findings may seem miraculous, the truth is anyone can reduce his or her body age. Many aging influences are at least partly within your control, and can be substantially affected by how you handle life's countless strains and pressures. If too harried to eat properly, you will not get the nourishment you need, and will be vulnerable to illness. If you cope with stress by smoking and drinking or taking tranquilizers, you are introducing more toxins into your body. And it is common knowledge that accidents are more likely to occur when people are tired, upset or in a hurry.

Eventually the biological damage from these factors weakens your body to the point that one or another degenerative disease surfaces. Fortunately, signs of premature aging almost always appear long before symptoms of acute illness. And the solution to counteracting these symptoms is much more within your control than you may think. Scientific evidence increasingly points to mental attitude. Just as outlook governs how a person handles major crises, so a person's state of mind controls the ability to deal with more routine tensions.

UNDERSTANDING STRESS

The body derives its energy from food. But how you use this energy is primarily the result of a bodily process called the stress reaction. The stress reaction mobilizes and channels your available strength to meet any challenge you face. So, in a sense, stress is actually a source of energy. How efficiently you use stress-energy will ultimately determine your day-to-day state of well-being and influence your rate of aging.

The stress reaction is a normal process your body goes through many times a day, as you deal with the fluctuating demands of your life. By triggering the release of certain hormones, stress produces a heightened state of body function that allows you to cope with or adapt to changing circumstances.

In its own right, stress is not good or bad. The chemical reaction is the same, whether it leaves you feeling exhilarated or exhausted. It may be that, one day, science detects a minor difference in the chemical composition of 'good' and 'bad' stress, but for now there is only one apparent difference: perception.

Stress you experience as positive is accompanied by a low level of uncertainty, and a high degree of choice. Some of the best things in life are extremely stressful — intense joy, deep love, sex, creativity.

On the other hand, people perceive stress as negative when they feel uncertain, ambivalent or powerless. Negative stress is stress you don't want, are unsure how to handle or feel unable to control — like getting stuck in traffic, getting fired, spraining your ankle. We refer to negative stress as distress.

The difference between people who generally perceive stress as good, and people who generally experience it as bad is this notion of stress-energy efficiency.

Fight or Flight: The Stress Reaction

Stress is a very primitive physical reaction that provides us with the energy either to fight or flee. It is a mechanism for adapting to unexpected events in the world, and is probably unchanged since the first humans walked the face of the earth millions of years ago.

Dr. Hans Selye, the father of modern stress research, identified three basic stages the body goes through each time it experiences a stress reaction: firstly alarm, secondly resistance or adaptation and thirdly exhaustion. This process is known as the general adaptation syndrome, or GAS.

The alarm stage — Our first response to change or danger is a general alarm. Your body perceives a stressor, something new or unusual that seems to represent a challenge or a threat. The stressor may be psychological (anger), physical (pain) or biological (illness).

Your hypothalamus, a gland responsible for maintaining homeostasis or functional balance in the body, triggers a series of chemical and electrical changes in your body.

In response, your body's metabolism, the rate at which you burn calories, speeds up. Your heart beats faster and your blood pressure rises. You begin to perspire. The lungs take in more air, your pupils dilate, your mouth goes dry, the hairs on your skin stand on end. You may experience the sensation of butterflies in your stomach. To some degree, you experience such feelings every time you are stressed.

Next, blood begins to flow away from peripheral areas in order to maximize the effectiveness of essential organs, such as the heart and lungs. As a result, skin begins to pale, and may become cold and clammy. The digestive system starts to shut down, which is why you may feel queasy. Blood also flows away from areas of your brain responsible for problem solving and information processing, impairing these faculties. And, because of the increased adrenaline flow, you start to have trouble concentrating and difficulty staying still.

While all these changes are designed to help you cope with stress, they also temporarily suppress your immune system.

The resistance phase — In the adaptation phase you are coping, successfully or not, with altered circumstances. This state will continue as long as heightened readiness or actual action seems necessary, which has a great deal to do with how you perceive the situation. Unfortunately, many people stay in the heightened stage long after a particular challenge has passed. The heart keeps pumping overtime and the muscles remain tense. People susceptible to prolonged stress reactions often complain they have trouble relaxing after a tough day or a big meeting. If you experience stress often, you may not be aware you are in a state of heightened resistance. It becomes a familiar plateau, upon which you are always poised for alarm.

The exhaustion stage — Exhaustion, the period of tiredness that follows, is an important part of the adaptation process. Once the threat has passed, the adrenal glands release cortisol, which reverses the stress reaction and returns the body to normal. The nervous system now sends calming messages throughout the body. Blood flows back to the skin surfaces, digestive tract and brain. The body relaxes, seizing the opportunity for much-needed rest and recuperation. But as a side effect of the release of cortisol, the immune system is once again suppressed.

Ideally, after the exhaustion phase, your body regains its equilibrium. You can short circuit the resistance phase by recognizing and regulating your stress reactions; essentially, choosing how to spend your stress-energy.

Distress

The longer and more intense a stress reaction, the more wear and tear it will inflict on your body, and the longer it will take your body to recuperate. People who spend too much time in the resistance phase often use caffeine or other stimulants to prolong it, long after their body says enough, and they frequently resort to drugs like alcohol to ease themselves into stage three.

Over time this can lead to distress. The immune system becomes compromised and you become more susceptible to a wide range of ailments. Everyone experiences distress from time to time. However, many of us are so used to its symptoms that we simply accept them as part of a demanding job, raising children or simply getting older.

From our research at the Canadian Institute of Stress we have identified five distinct phases of chronic distress, which nearly everyone passes through as tensions escalate. You may find that you experience several phases at once, that you get stuck in a particular phase or that you tend to cycle through all five over and over again.

Phase one: chronic mental or physical fatigue — Early in this stage, you need coffee or strong tea to get going in the morning and probably several more to get you through the day. Even so, you experience low energy in the afternoon. When you get home from work, you want to collapse. At night you tend to sleep poorly and wake up tense, or sleep soundly but don't feel refreshed. Over time, collapse seems to hit you earlier and earlier, until one morning you can barely drag yourself out of bed.

Phase two: interpersonal problems and withdrawal — In the second phase of distress, problems with co-workers, family and friends surface. You withdraw from contact with others, and become suspicious of the people around you or feel hostile toward them. As you walk around with a chip on your shoulder, your boiling point gets lower and lower, and you become angry or upset over trivial events.

You spend less time on relationships, putting less energy into them and getting less out. You may seem to spend the same amount of time with your spouse but increasingly find you are living separate lives in the same space. Your sense of satisfaction and support diminishes, and increasingly you withdraw into yourself. Small problems become insurmountable.

Phase three: emotional turbulence — In phase three, the simmer of phase two becomes an almost constant boil. The churning cauldron of emotions inside is no longer mainly directed outward. You become filled with self doubt, and unable to focus, arrange priorities or make decisions. Interpersonal problems become even more pronounced, and emotional anchors and relationships more tenuous. Your ability to maintain emotional balance diminishes. You become easily depressed or find yourself blowing up without warning. Your reaction is out of proportion to the event that caused it. More and more you teeter between extremes; you are either keyed up or depressed. Your performance at work suffers noticeably.

Phase four: chronic physical discomfort — At this point your body starts to inform you loudly that you are spending far too much time in a state of constant vigilance. Chronic muscle tension, particularly in the neck and shoulder area, lower back and across the forehead becomes the norm. You may find you clench your teeth or grind at night, or that you are subject to chronic headaches that escalate to migraines when you finally do try to relax.

Phase five: stress-related illness — This phase of exhaustion has been compared to extreme old age. Research shows that stress-related illness is synonymous with rapidly accelerated aging. Traditionally, doctors have tried to help by treating the disease, but increasingly it is being understood that you also need to address the underlying cause, and prescribe behavioural changes.

We at the Canadian Institute of Stress believe all five phases of distress are indicators of accelerated aging. Our body age study showed that distress can be reversed, and body age lowered, through a combination of lifestyle changes uniquely tailored to each individual.

REGULATING STRESS

The creative potential of stress-energy is evident in the amazing feats men and women have accomplished, often in extraordinary circumstances. The solider in battle who saves the life of a peer; the athlete who breaks a world record. Assuming you have a healthy diet and are physically fit, the key to having stress-energy available when you need it is not to waste it when you don't.

Every person has an optimum operating level; a function of age, nutrition, fitness and genetics. Every athlete who has trained for a big game, or any executive who has prepared for a big meeting, knows that performance levels rise as the expenditure of stress-energy increases, up to the point of maximum efficiency. After this, you get a diminished return on your investment of energy, and performance starts to decline.

It may be a crisis that puts you over the edge or one additional small stressor that tips the balance. Whatever the trigger, it is at this point that you are likely to smash your car or sprain your ankle. Insurance companies are well aware that six months following a marriage breakup, the chance of having an automobile accident doubles.

Before you can learn to stay out of the danger zone, you need to acquire the skills to monitor your position on your personal stress performance curve. You need to be able to identify whether stress is providing the edge you need, or if it is interfering with your ability to handle a situation well.

The Stress Master

People who cycle through the five phases of distress are gambling with their well-being. The workaholic is one example of a chronic stress gambler. For most workaholics it is not really work they are addicted to. It is the beta endorphins the body produces during the stress reaction; hormones that create a feeling of exhilaration. Like a drug addict, they need more and more to maintain the high.

Many people who are very successful are not workaholics but stress masters. They may work long hours and use a great deal of stress-energy, but they are focused and efficient. As a result, their return on the stress-energy investment is high. Their satisfactions buffer them from experiencing distress. They also know how to relax, even in the midst of a tension-producing day.

Mastering stress allows you to exert conscious control over primarily reflexive body functions. In essence, it allows you to make stress work for you and to experience stress as something positive. The body constantly seeks to return to a steady healthy state. As long as you don't undermine it, the body will always strive for maximum efficiency. To achieve a steady healthy state you must first understand your stress type.

What is Your Stress Type?

A stress type is a profile of a lifestyle prone to accelerated aging. Through our body age study we identified six types. Each is inefficient at managing stress, but in a different way. All people exhibit some of the traits of each type, but will tend to have one or two stress types that are predominant.

The Speed Freak

We all know speed freaks, or people with Type-A personalities — whether they are constant speeders or people who go through manic periods. Unable to slow down, these individuals are always two steps ahead, even of themselves. Frequently, they are seemingly successful people.

But, although speed freaks are people on the move, they often don't have a clear idea of where they're going or why they're heading there so fast. They work and play with great intensity, apparently unable to distinguish between the important and less important. They are extremely impatient when waiting — in line, in traffic, for a friend who's late. At work, at home, at play, they tend to try to do two or three things at once. In fact, speed freaks often have trouble simply sitting still and find it difficult to slow down for others.

Fitful sleepers, speed freaks may rise early, charged with adrenaline before they're fully rested. They may be subject to periods of total collapse but tend to hide them from even their most intimate circle. Apart from these occasional let downs they do not seem to know how to relax. They must have endless projects to fill their leisure time.

More than any other stress type, speed freaks waste stress-energy needlessly by keeping their bodies in a heightened state of alertness. When additional energy is required, they quickly become overstressed. This takes its toll physically. Studies show that people with a high susceptibility to heart attacks or other cardiovascular problems are often speed freaks.

The Basket Case

People who fall into this category are often tired even before the day begins. At work, the basket case is constantly fighting low energy; simply functioning takes an act of will. Consequently, the basket case often burdens co-workers and friends, who must pitch in to help.

For this stress type physical symptoms abound, from migraine headaches to tight aching muscles — all arising from no specific medical cause. If a doctor suggests more exercise, the basket case begs off, citing fatigue. These people are especially prone to colds, flu and allergies. Not surprisingly, conversation for the basket case consists largely of complaints about ill health. Such behavior can trigger a downward spiral, leading to job loss and the breakup of relationships.

Being physically unfit is at the root of the basket case's difficulties. He or she simply does not have the stamina to respond to stressors in a healthy way. At first glance, however, people suffering from this stress type may not appear unfit.

The Cliff Walker

As the name implies, the cliff walker is someone who lives on the edge, entertaining a lifestyle of indulgence and self abuse. Along with the speed freak, he or she is the most likely candidate for a fatal heart attack in his or her 30s or 40s. Cliff walkers are susceptible to a host of other illnesses and complaints, ranging from migraine headaches to arthritis.

Not surprisingly, cliff walkers have poor health and dietary habits, such as smoking, drinking to excess and using tranquilizers and stimulants. Often they are overweight and unable to stick to either a diet or an exercise program. Under such duress, it is only a matter of time before the weakest system fails and the cliff walker topples off the precipice.

The Drifter

In our study, drifters fell into two main categories: people who never seemed to have found a goal or direction or, alternatively, people going through a mid-life crisis, questioning their goals and the sacrifices they've made to achieve them. Retirees and homemakers whose children have grown up sometimes exhibit such tendencies.

Whether the crisis comes in mid-life or at some other time, the typical drifter feels blocked from becoming the ideal person he or she dreams of being. Most people experience such feelings at some point, doubting for a time the personal value of what they have accomplished. But when these life crises continue for years, they can wreak havoc, profoundly affecting productivity and personal relationships. As the gap between reality and ideals becomes more acutely felt, it can lead to deep depression, personal paralysis and an impulsive life change, with sometime disastrous consequences.

Drifters waste stress-energy through psychological uncertainty. They never apply themselves wholeheartedly to any one job or life project; haphazardly approaching many different challenges instead, undermining themselves through self doubt. They aren't sure what they want; they only know it isn't what they already have.

The Worry Wart

Naturally, a certain amount of worrying serves a useful function, helping us anticipate and prepare for problems that lie ahead. But for worry warts, anxiety about the future and anguish over the past have virtually taken over. Worry warts create problems that aren't there, and make small concerns into life-and-death issues. They expend so much energy worrying about themselves — their health, jobs, relationships — they have little vigor left for living and working.

A worry wart is the sort of person about whom friends say, "If he weren't worrying, I'd be worried." As might be expected, relationships suffer from this continual anxiety. And the worry wart's career is likely to be characterized by many promising starts that soon fizzle out. Ironically, worry warts believe that anxiety is either the price of success or a barrier to achievement.

The Loner

Although loners do not necessarily live alone, they do tend to avoid social contacts. Even in a marriage, loners engage in minimal communication. Consequently, they feel isolated most of the time, even in a crowd and especially at a social gathering of friends.

In essence, loners do not know how to establish intimate relationships. Quite often the few friends such people have, perhaps from high school or college days, gradually fade away and no new ones take their place. Over time, loners forget how to conduct conversations of a personal nature. The workplace also offers little consolation. Although loners can be single minded and successful in their careers, they derive decreasing satisfaction from them. In desperation, they become solo drinkers, seeking comfort within themselves.

DEALING WITH STRESS

Now that you have an idea of your dominant stress type(s), you can choose the specific anti-aging skills that will be most helpful to you, and write your own prescription for change. Through our study we found five interventions to be the most potent for combating aging. These are values/goals clarification, effective relaxation, self-affirming communication, high-performance nutrition and exercise.

For some, the prescription will follow common sense. For example, if your dominant stress type is cliff walker, a type who suffers from numerous bodily ailments, your primary intervention is improved nutrition.

Some of our recommendations, however, are counter-intuitive. For the loner, for instance, we found that improving communication skills was not the most constructive place to start. To tackle this area would have meant altering deeply entrenched attitudes and habits; something very difficult to do.

Instead, loners seem to achieve the best results by concentrating first on values/goals clarification. In the process of doing so, they come to see that obtaining their goals often means interacting positively with other people. Understanding this then enables loners to tackle the thorny area of relationships.

If your own prescription means starting with an anti-aging skill that does not seem to address your stress type directly, don't be concerned. Eventually you will be ready to modify the specific behavior that is causing you distress.

Values/Goals Clarification
As it happens, values/goals clarification — which teaches techniques for determining what is important to you — ranked a surprising first overall, ahead of the physical relaxation techniques that are usually emphasized in stress management.

It may be that defining values leads to greater acceptance of self. Because such positive feelings tend to enhance

Prescription Wheel

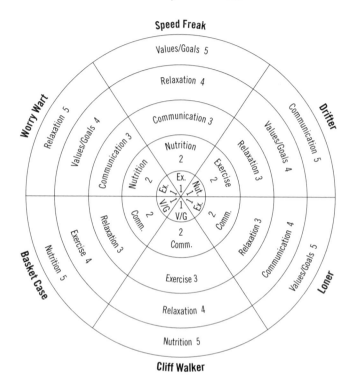

a person's health, it makes sense that this technique would be particularly powerful. Or it could be that in order to use stress-energy efficiently, you need a clear sense of priorities. Only then can you decide where you want to invest your precious capital of energy and time.

There is growing evidence that people who survive highly disturbing experiences, such as the concentration camps of World War II, are those who have a deep rooted sense of values. These inform day-to-day behaviour, helping people achieve a sense of control against seemingly insurmountable odds.

Relaxation

Effective relaxation ranked second in terms of helping people improve their stress-energy efficiency. This is because relaxation alone won't prevent people from returning to destructive patterns but, combined with other anti-aging skills, it is extremely useful. Learning effective techniques can help you pace yourself as you practice other skills.

Communication

Self-affirming communication ranked third in our study and is a potent force in reducing body age as well as increasing vitality in loners and drifters. In its most essential form, assertive, or self-affirming, communication means revealing your self to another person. It emphasizes the confident putting forward of needs, opinion, claims and rights — while remaining sensitive to the feelings and positions of others. Self-affirming communication strikes a balance between speaking and listening, between sending and receiving.

The benefits of self-affirming communication are considerable. Since relationships are the biggest source of uncertainty in most people's lives, improved communication dramatically increases confidence, lowering stress. Assertive communication removes roadblocks in relationships. And, at its best, it enables you to truly perceive another person's point of view. As you acquire better communication skills, you'll find all your relationships improving.

Exercise

Exercise only ranked fourth as an anti-aging skill. Although it is important, it may be overrated by experts in stress and health. In fact, a growing body of data suggest that the effectiveness of corporate fitness programs stems at least as much from the subsidiary effects as from the physical routines themselves — feelings of camaraderie with fellow participants, for example. Like relaxation, it is quite potent in combination with other life skills.

Nutrition

Although proper nutrition clearly has great potential for promoting optimum health and vitality, it ranked last as an anti-aging strategy. However, we then found that when a broad based vitamin/mineral supplement was added to sensible dietary habits, the skill soared to second place.

In part, this may stem from the fact that sound nutrition is relatively easy to teach, but very difficult for most people to follow. Also, the same foods can vary in vitamin and mineral content. There is some evidence as well that chemical additives have an adverse effect on nutrition. Because of this dichotomy in the ranking of nutrition, we concluded that a vitamin/mineral supplement is essential to an anti-aging program.

Our study clearly showed that success in one area influences success in another. Think of your prescription as emergency first aid for someone in distress. A lifelong approach to rejuvenation is to become an expert in all five of the life skills, which will ultimately make you a stress master. When you accomplish that, who knows what heights of vitality are possible for you.

Sleep

By Dr. Colin Shapiro, PhD

Sleep and Alertness Clinic

Dawn, a 57-year-old retired writer, never had trouble sleeping. She fell asleep and woke at the same time each day with little effort, and generally faced each day feeling rested and refreshed. But over the past five years she noticed her sleep habits changing. Increasingly, she found herself getting tired earlier and earlier, to the point that she could hardly keep her eyes open after nine o'clock. Although she could fall asleep easily enough, after a few hours she would wake and have a hard time falling back to sleep. By four or five o'clock in the morning she was wide awake.

Changes in the way we sleep are a normal part of aging, though perhaps an under-reported one. As we age, our ability to sleep through the night decreases and the prevalence of sleep disorders increases. Like Dawn, you may fall asleep and wake earlier, your night may be interrupted by frequent awakenings or you may simply not feel refreshed after a night's sleep, even when you get eight or nine hours of slumber. If you have a medical disease or chronic illness, such as cardiovascular disease or diabetes, and are taking medications for your condition, your likelihood of experiencing sleep problems increases all the more.

Unfortunately, few of us get the recommended seven to nine hours of sleep a night. Today, many people tend to see sleep as an inconvenience; a nuisance that gets in the way of their work and life. The National Sleep Foundation reports that the national average for sleep is six hours 54 minutes. That number dips even lower during the work week, when we are more likely to give work obligations priority over a good night's sleep. This means that nearly half of North Americans are not getting enough sleep, and that by the time we reach middle age we may be in a state of chronic sleep deprivation.

Despite this overwhelming evidence of sleeplessness, few people report having sleep problems to their doctor. Only five percent of people with insomnia visit a doctor specifically to discuss their sleep complaint, and a mere 25 percent bring it up during the course of a visit for another purpose. The majority never mention their sleep problems at all, to the detriment of their sleep satisfaction and often that of their partner as well.

To age smart, we need to be a great deal more sleep savvy. Sleep is not an optional activity; it is as essential to life as water and food, and has numerous health benefits.

THE NATURAL CYCLES OF SLEEP

Our 24-hour sleep-wake cycle is governed by *circadian rhythms*. Controlled by the sun, circadian rhythms keep the body alert during daylight hours, and help it to relax when night falls. This inner clock will even awaken you when you forget to set your alarm. Circadian rhythms also affect hormones and influence body temperature.

Within our daily sleep-wake cycle, there is a regular pattern of sleep, known as *sleep architecture*. Based on research, we know that the sleep architecture of a healthy night's slumber has a progressive pattern of incrementally deeper sleep, which repeats several times each night.

During the night you cycle through two different sleep states; REM and Non-REM sleep. Non-REM sleep is divided into three stages, characterized by increasingly slower brain waves. The first stage, light sleep, is a dream-less light doze. In the second stage, intermediate or midlevel sleep, brain-wave activity becomes unsettled, with irregular patterns and spikes. This is followed by semi-deep and deep sleep, marked by slow, high-amplitude delta waves. Deep sleep mostly takes place in the first third of the night and appears to be quite important to health.

Once you cycle through these three stages, you typically return to stage two (intermediate sleep) and then proceed to REM, the rapid eye movement stage where dreaming takes place. Brain-wave activity during REM is in the beta range, a state of full alertness when you're awake, which may explain why dreams can seem and feel so realistic. Most REM sleep takes place in the last third of the night.

Sleep and Aging

As we age, there are predicable changes in our sleep architecture. Although there is a small decrease in duration of sleep with aging, there is unquestionably a 'catastrophic' decline in the amount of deep (restorative) sleep. This decline is thought to begin in the third decade of life, with a steady decline each decade thereafter. When you are in your 20s, for instance, 20 percent of the night is comprised of slow-wave (deep) sleep. At 40 years of age slow-wave sleep declines to ten percent, and at 60 years it falls to five percent. Furthermore, the actual slow waves (the indicators of deep sleep) have smaller amplitude. At the same time as this pronounced decline in deep sleep, there is a marked increase in the lightest stage of sleep; stage one.

Sleep-wake patterns also change with aging. Compared with younger adults, total sleep, as well as sleep efficiency — the percentage of in-bed time spent asleep — decrease as we age, falling by as much as 30 percent after age 60. At the same time, night-time awakenings increase. This means that if you spend seven hours in bed, only 4.9 to 5.6 hours are actually spent sleeping. Together, these changes predispose to lighter, more fragmented and less restorative sleep. What's more, the sleep-wake cycle commonly shifts to earlier hours with age. This can result in awakening around three or four in the morning without being able to return to sleep, as well as sleepiness at seven or eight in the evening.

Paradoxically, the older we get the more time we often spend in bed, as if trying to accumulate the extra sleep we feel we need. This is counterproductive. Having high sleep efficiency is a key component in determining how satisfying we believe our sleep to be. For example, if you spend five and a half hours in bed, and sleep five of those hours, you will feel more satisfied than if you sleep six hours, and spend eight and a half hours in bed.

There are also hormonal changes that occur with aging that affect sleep quality. During deep sleep, adults secrete the majority of their human growth hormone (HGH). HGH is important for building bone and muscle mass and discouraging the storage of fat, but invariably declines with aging. By age 50, men are often critically short on deep sleep and, as a result, may lose muscle mass and gain fat. Secretions of the hormone melatonin may also decline in some, and become more erratic. Instead of a spike of excretion at 10:00 pm, the peak is dampened and spread over many hours. We refer to these hormonal changes as endopause.

Benefits of Sleep

Getting a good night's sleep will do more than keep you alert the next day. Many studies have shown that individuals who sleep an average of seven to nine hours a night have the longest life expectancy. This is because sleep has a number of health benefits, giving us the chance to maintain and repair our bodies and minds.

Memory — As we age, we often attribute memory slips to the inevitable effects of aging on our brains when, in fact, insufficient sleep may be the culprit. Although it is not clear exactly how, sleep seems to help the brain consolidate and organize memory. But if you don't get enough, memory can be significantly impaired. The longer you are sleep-deprived and run a sleep debt (the amount of sleep you 'owe' in order to return to baseline health and performance), the more frequent and pervasive forgetfulness can be. Get enough sleep, and you will find it easier to recall names and to remember just where you left the car keys.

Mood — The most potent effects of sleep deprivation are on behaviour. Sleep is regulated in the same area of the brain that controls mood, body temperature and hormones — the hypothalamus. Also known as the emotion centre, the hypothalamus is happiest when you've had plenty of sleep. In fact, mood is even more dramatically impaired by sleep deprivation than is physical performance or mental function. A number of studies have shown that depression is one of the biggest risk factors for insomnia, and vice-versa. People who, for whatever reason, do not sleep well are more at risk for developing depression. Conversely, people who feel good emotionally generally sleep better.

Immunity — The immune system is markedly affected by sleep loss. Studies have shown that the response to the flu vaccine is affected by the amount of sleep that you had during the days prior to vaccination. If you have not had enough sleep when you are immunized, the amount of antibody that you build may be reduced by as much as 50 percent. This is because your body translates sleep deprivation as stress, and responds by releasing stress hormones that can weaken immune responses, leaving you vulnerable to invading germs and antigens. (See Chapter Six for more on stress).

Accident prevention — We are all well aware of the dangers of driving drunk, but what about driving sleep-deprived?

In an Australian study, it was shown that sleep loss is comparable to the level of impairment that you experience from alcohol. In fact, a number of people that are on the road have a sleep debt that puts them at the same level of impairment as if they had more than the legal limit of alcohol in their blood.

Owls and Larks

Although we are essentially programmed to sleep during the night and be active during the day, some people have a marked morning or evening preference. Researchers believe that owls — people who like to stay up late — and larks — people who like to get up early — have their body clocks set to different schedules. The body clock, also described as the body's circadian rhythm, controls sleep-wake patterns by regulating body temperature and hormones such as melatonin and cortisol.

In most people, melatonin rises just before going to bed and drops just after waking up. Cortisol peaks just before waking up. And body temperature hits the lowest point around the middle of a night's sleep. In larks, however, these hormonal fluctuations and temperature rhythms occur earlier than they do for most people, so they get tired earlier in the evening and perform best in the morning. This may be due to a genetic factor, or due to social or biological factors. For example, some people may become lark-like because they have a two-hour commute to work.

On the other hand, people who are owls experience these hormonal fluctuations later in the day, and may just be hitting their stride as their work day is ending. When required to function on a 'normal' schedule, these people can end up sleep-deprived due to insomnia. For this reason, larks tend to have fewer problems due to their sleep habits, though their social lives may suffer. However, when larks have to work at night, as shift workers do, they find that they tire much earlier than their peers.

Although it might take a bit of doing, most owls and larks can reset their body clocks by following the sleep recommendations at the end of this chapter.

SLEEP PROBLEMS

There is a strong correlation between increasing age and the likelihood of a sleep disorder. Daytime sleepiness and finding it hard to wake up in the morning are the most obvious signs of a sleep shortage. Other telltale signs include dropping off in front of the TV, drowsiness during long meetings, needing lots of coffee to stay awake and droopy eyes while driving.

Insomnia

Insomnia is the most common sleep complaint of older adults, affecting more than 35 million North Americans. The good news is that, for most people, insomnia is not a disease that causes sleeplessness, but rather a symptom of physical, psychological or environmental factors that are keeping them awake. These most commonly include emotions like stress, worry or excitement, schedule or time zone changes and a poor sleeping environment. We all experience varying degrees of such disruptions at different times in our lives, but some people are more sensitive to these variables than others.

Sleep-Disordered Breathing

Also known as sleep apnea, this condition occurs when your body briefly forgets to, or can't, breathe while you sleep, causing you to wake up, sometimes countless times a night. The prevalence of sleep apnea is strongly associated with obesity, and increases with age, in its mild form affecting 30 to 50 percent of middle-aged men and 47 percent of post-menopausal women. The most common form of sleep apnea is associated with obstruction to airflow during sleep, due to collapse of the upper airway at the back of the throat. Symptoms of sleep apnea include loud snoring or gasping for air many times a night, daytime sleepiness, impaired daytime performance, morning headaches and/or sexual problems. Few people know that they're waking up gasping for air many times a night, but the stress on their body, not to mention that of the person sleeping next to them, can be severe. Fortunately, sleep apnea can be successfully treated with a machine that aids breathing, or relieved by oral devices or surgery.

Restless Legs Syndrome

Restless legs syndrome (RLS) — twitching or restlessness that prevents you from falling asleep — and periodic limb movements in sleep (PLMS) — movements and awakening from sleep because of leg twitching — affect as many as 35 percent of people 65 years and older. In RLS, pre-sleep leg discomfort and the urge to move the legs can result in difficulty getting to sleep. Today, experts estimate that as many as eight percent of people in the United States have this neurological condition. While the cause of RLS syndrome is unknown, a family history of the condition is seen in approximately 50 percent of people, suggesting a genetic form of the disorder.

PLMS involves leg kicks every 20 to 40 seconds during the night, which result in repeated arousals, unrefreshing sleep and daytime sleepiness. Like sleep apnea, these movements can wake you up again and again during the night without your knowledge. If you suffer from either of these conditions, seek medical help. Research has shown certain vitamins and supplements may help.

A GOOD NIGHT'S SLEEP

While the occasional disrupted night is normal, ongoing sleep difficulties, especially if they occur more than a couple of nights per week, merit intervention. Whether you face age-related sleep challenges, insomnia or a medical condition that keeps you awake, there are many things you can do to improve your sleep.

Keep a Sleep Diary

The best way to evaluate the health and quality of your sleep is to pay close attention to your sleep patterns, and to the way you feel throughout the entire day. Any drowsiness in the daytime means you have a significant sleep debt. Often our perceptions of our sleep habits are a far cry from the way we actually sleep, so, to get a true idea of your current sleep adequacy, track your sleeping patterns over a week or two. Besides sleep and awakening times and daytime functioning, your sleep diary should include the timing and amount of any medication, caffeine and alcohol use.

Get out in the Sun
Our body's circadian rhythms start to weaken with age, requiring more light to keep them synchronized. This can be easily retrained by increasing your exposure to natural daylight. Open the curtains during the day. Position your desk near a window or use a lightbook at work, or wherever you spend the most time. Most importantly, get out in natural sunlight as often as you can. Just like your skin, your eyes can soak up the sun's rays even on cloudy days.

Exercise
One of the most effective ways to get a good night's sleep is to increase your activity during the day. Daily exercise, even if only for a short period, tends to be 'sleep protective' at any age, increasing the amount of deep, slow-wave sleep. To get the sleep-promoting benefits of exercise, time your workout no later than three to four hours before bedtime. Exercise too close to bedtime is invigorating and can make it harder to fall asleep.

Relax
It may seem obvious, but being able to relax will go a long way towards improving your quality of sleep. There are a number of techniques proven to promote a sense of relaxation:

- Alternatively tense and relax each of the major muscle groups
- Imagine your body parts being immersed in warm water or covered with warm blankets
- Take a warm bath before bed; the temperature elevation can help induce deep sleep

Make Your Bedroom a Sleep Sanctuary

In many cases your sleeping environment could be contributing to your sleep problem. Make certain you have a comfortable bed and a bedroom that is conducive to sleep. Block out unnecessary light by getting eyeshades or blackout curtains. Adjust the room's temperature to a moderate level.

Look also at the light sources in your bedroom. Night lights and alarm clocks are some of the worst culprits. Not only do some LED displays emit enough light to fool you into thinking it's morning all night long, but also the temptation to check the time during the night worries your tired mind about how late or early it is — stimulation you don't need. People with insomnia should turn the display at an angle, so they can still see the time but more of the light is directed away from their eyes.

Finally, reduce noise in your bedroom. People often think that sound doesn't bother their sleep. Research clearly shows that is not the case. A study of people who lived near a noisy airport found that they averaged an hour less sleep each night than those living in quiet neighbourhoods. If street noise is a problem in your area, look for drapes that block sound as well as light. Add carpeting and wall hangings to help absorb the sound. Wear earplugs, or use a white noise machine. For the same reason, if you have a TV in your room, move it. Watching television in bed de-conditions your mind from sleep, and over stimulates the body and brain. Ultimately, your bed should be reserved for sleep and sex.

Take a Time-Out

People with insomnia often come to associate bedtime rituals and features of the sleep environment with difficulty sleeping, thereby perpetuating the sleep problem. The same holds true for chronic worriers, who are kept awake at night by anxiety. If you cannot sleep after about 20 minutes, either upon initially retiring or after awakening during the night, get out of bed and do something relaxing, and slightly boring, until you get sleepy again (i.e. no stimulating TV programs). This can be repeated as necessary. The aim is to associate the sleep environment with falling asleep quickly.

Practice Good Sleep Hygiene

Good sleep hygiene, a set of habits that promote sound sleep, is especially important for people with sleep problems. Sleep hygiene involves commonsense principles, aimed at ensuring that your behaviours and your bedroom environment are conducive to night-time sleep.

- *Maintain a regular schedule* — A regular bed- and wake-time is the cornerstone of good sleep hygiene. As we age, most people's internal clocks become more inflexible. To help your biological clock work with and not against you, maintain a regular bedtime and wake time, seven days a week; even if you had a bad night's sleep the night before. Experience shows that it may take several nights of bad sleep for the body to begin to achieve good and regular sleep.
- *Use your bed for sleep* — Because excessive time in bed can perpetuate sleep problems like insomnia, time in bed should be restricted to equal the total sleep time previously recorded in your sleep diary. Rising time is based on your usual schedule, and bedtime set accordingly, but not so as to allow less than 4.5 hours of sleep. Once you are sleeping efficiently (i.e. sleep time =

time in bed), you can retire 15 minutes earlier. Adjust your bedtime up or down by 15 minutes per week to maintain sleep efficiency.

- *No naps* — Napping during the day is shown to exacerbate poor-quality sleep. Even if you feel tired, curtail naps and bed rest. If you must nap, keep it brief and nap earlier in the day.

- *Avoid caffeine after lunch* — Often when we can't sleep and feel fatigued during the day, we drink coffee (or colas) to keep awake. Too much caffeine, particularly late in the day, will keep you up during the night. To prevent caffeine from disrupting your sleep, drink no more than two cups of coffee a day, and avoid drinking caffeine after noontime.

- *Avoid nicotine* — Like coffee, smoking is a stimulant, which will make it harder for you to fall asleep and will shorten the time you sleep during the night. If you must smoke, do not do so before bedtime or during the night.

- *Limit alcohol* — Many people drink alcohol to try to help them sleep. While alcohol may help you fall asleep, it will actually have the opposite effect later in the night, when it wakes you up. Furthermore, with continued drinking the sleep-inducing effect disappears.

- *Don't eat a heavy meal before bed* — If you're hungry, try a light snack such as a few crackers or a slice of toast. Better yet, try a few slices of turkey, a banana or a glass of warm milk about an hour before bedtime. These foods contain L-tryptophan, a natural sleep enhancer.

Sleep Hygiene Rules

- Engage in quiet activities and avoid stimulating activity just before bedtime

- Do not go to bed until you are sleepy

- Reserve the bed for sleeping and sex; do not read or watch TV in bed

- Get up at the same time each morning and go to bed at the same time each night, including weekends

- Avoid naps if they disrupt sleep the following night; otherwise, limit them to the early afternoon

- Get regular exercise and enjoy regular social activity (but avoid strenuous activity after 6:00 pm)

- Eliminate or minimize alcohol use; do not drink alcohol within two hours of bedtime

- Eliminate or minimize caffeine use; do not consume caffeine after 4:00 pm. (Especially sensitive individuals should avoid caffeine after noon)

- Eliminate or minimize smoking; do not smoke within four hours of bedtime

- Avoid heavy meals before bedtime; a light carbohydrate snack, such as milk, banana or turkey, which contain tryptophan, may promote sleep.

- The sleep environment should be comfortable, without being too warm, and should admit minimal light and noise

Supplements

There is some evidence that certain supplements may be sleep-promoting.

Melatonin — Melatonin is a nocturnally secreted hormone involved in regulating circadian rhythms. Its secretion is disrupted with aging. Melatonin is also a potent free-radical scavenger. As melatonin levels drop with aging, the accumulation of free radicals may promote anatomic and functional degeneration, thereby contributing to sleep dysfunction. While data are conflicting, a recent systematic review suggests that melatonin supplementation may be beneficial in some older adults. However, because melatonin is a hormone, it should not be taken without having an appropriate test.

Tryptophan — Some people prefer to take this sleep-promoting substance, which is found in foods such as milk, cheese, banana, tuna and turkey, over other hypnotics. There is evidence that certain individuals' sleep disturbances respond to tryptophan supplementation. However, data are conflicting and further research is required.

E
I
G
H
T

Sex

By Dr. Frank Sommers, MD, FRCPC

Psychiatrist and Medical Sex Therapist

Sandra and Pat, married for 25 years, had always enjoyed an active sex life. Even with the stress of raising three children on Pat's single income and managing the family's hectic schedule, they still made time for intimacy. But over the past few years their sex life had become more sporadic. At 50 years of age the effects of arthritis and menopause had taken their toll on Sandra's body. What she once enjoyed in the bedroom was now uncomfortable, sometimes even painful. Feeling old before her time, she increasingly found excuses to avoid sex. Hurt by her decreased interest, Pat interpreted her actions as a loss of interest in him and stopped initiating sexual activity. Increasingly the couple was feeling the distance between them.

The old stereotype of losing interest in sex as we age has long been dispelled. Studies show that interest in and enjoyment of sex continues well into later life, with many men and women remaining sexually active well into their 70s and beyond. Unfortunately others will short change their sex life. Misunderstandings about the body changes they may be undergoing as they age lead some people to put unnecessary limitations on their sexual relationships, or to stop having sex altogether. If you avoid sex with your partner because you don't think it can be enjoyable after menopause, or fear that your partner is losing interest in you because he or she no longer responds to your advances, chances are you are selling yourself short on one of life's most basic pleasures and fundamental bonding experiences.

As with other parts of the body, age has an impact on sexual function. With each decade after age 40 come anticipatable changes in your ability to respond to sexual stimuli. Clearly understanding these changes and then communicating them to your partner is the key to maintaining an active and fulfilling sex life as you age. Sometimes this is easier said than done. Like Sandra and Pat, many couples are reluctant to discuss subtle changes in their ability to function sexually. They may be embarrassed by what they perceive as sexual dysfunction when in fact they are just undergoing the natural and normal changes of age. The result is an escalating and ultimately self-defeating cycle that can potentially lead to abstinence, diminished quality of life, depression, extra-relationship affairs or separation.

Sexual difficulties can begin as minor changes and escalate into more complex problems if not addressed at an early stage. By the time most men turn 50 they will experience an inability to sustain an erection at least occasionally and, as they age, will find it can happen increasingly often. Women after menopause often lose their ability to self-lubricate and, if no intervention takes place, will find sex uncomfortable. Unrecognized, these types of sexual difficulties can lead to feelings of failure and loss of self-esteem. These feelings may be compounded by a partner's reaction of disappointment or anger.

The good news is that, with a little work and understanding, most sexual difficulties are easily manageable. But the earlier you start the better. Sexuality is like a sensitive flower. It has to be carefully tended and nurtured. This is best done when you are developing your relationship as a couple, and becomes increasingly important as you enter middle age, when you are more vulnerable to physical infirmities and weight gain.

AGE AND THE SEXUAL RESPONSE CYCLE

Though you may not think of sex as a prearranged sequence of events, there are five predictable phases that every person cycles through when achieving an orgasm. This process is known as the sexual response cycle and includes desire, arousal, plateau (the peak of arousal), orgasm and resolution phases. Understanding these phases and the effect age has on them can help demystify the changes in sexual function you may be experiencing now or down the road.

Desire Phase
We've all experienced times of heightened or diminished levels of sexual desire. When we fall in love, sexual desire can be at its most intense, while a bout of depression can

kill it altogether. Most people do not expect to maintain the libido they had in their 20s into their retirement years, but that does not mean you should expect sexual desire to dry up like a spring creek in the winter. The effect of aging on sexual desire varies greatly from person to person, depending on general and mental health as well as the state of a relationship.

It is well known that hormone levels are linked to sexual desire. In men, testosterone levels begin to decline at age 50 and continue to weaken steadily throughout later life, thus diminishing sexual desire. For both genders, DHEA levels begin to decline in the 30s and continue steadily thereafter, reaching quite low levels by age 60. If you are on medications to treat a chronic illness, it is likely that your androgen levels have been affected, which may decrease genital and breast sensitivity.

Desire can also be influenced by various environmental, psychological, cultural and physiologic processes. Life stressors can either begin or worsen at mid-life. Issues such as retirement, job loss, diminished income, divorce, unresolved anger, death of friends and family and illness can all lead to diminished desire. Studies show that financial stress is particularly detrimental. As life becomes increasingly expensive, worry over bills, children's education and old age can significantly impair sexual desire, function and libido. And, because desire and activity go hand in hand, the less sex you have, the less likely you are to desire it.

The final, but perhaps most important, influence on sexual desire is how you feel about your relationship with your partner. Like a house, relationships have an infrastructure. On getting together, a couple has a window of opportunity to establish a good foundation that will stand the passage of time. If that doesn't happen (i.e. they do not communicate their desires, concerns, etc.) there may be serious problems down the road. In many cases, lifelong psychological conflicts heighten as people age. Left unchecked these conflicts will eventually develop into resentment, which kills desire in a relationship. There will inevitably be irritants in every relationship — frustration, annoyance and anger. If dealt with regularly, these irritants will not destroy desire. But if left to fester, they will not only deprive people of energy and joie de vivre, but will also prevent the relationship from moving forward and may lead to depression, which can be very insidious. Like resentment, depression can take over a person or a relationship, enveloping it like a fog, and destroying sexual desire.

Arousal and Plateau Phases

In the arousal phase of the sexual response cycle, blood flow increases to the genitals, causing vaginal lubrication and penile erection, and peaks during the plateau phase at the height of arousal. These two phases rely on an intact parasympathetic and sympathetic nervous and vascular system, as well as the presence of desire. As we age, subtle changes in the peripheral nerves, blood vessels and muscle tissue can impair the body's ability to pump blood to the sexual organs. In men, erections may not be as hard, last as long or be as sensitive as they once were. In women, lubrication may become an issue as estrogen levels drop with menopause, leading to a reduction in sexual responsiveness.

Orgasm

The capacity to achieve orgasm is maintained with age. Many women remain capable of achieving orgasms, even multiple orgasms, near peak levels well into their senior years. For men, age tends to have a greater impact. Orgasms may become less frequent and vigorous for men, but will be as pleasurable as before. In both cases, achieving orgasm may entail a little more effort. Because genital sensitivity is reduced with age, men and women may require more direct physical stimulation in order to climax.

Resolution Phase

The final phase, resolution, involves a rush of blood away from the genitals and a reduction in heart rate, respiration and blood pressure. Resolution occurs more rapidly with age for both sexes, but is more pronounced in older men. Following orgasm, detumescence (loss of swelling) occurs rapidly, and the refractory period, or the amount of time that must pass before a man is capable of another ejaculation, significantly increases with age.

GENDER-SPECIFIC PROBLEMS IN SEXUAL FUNCTION

Within the general decline in sexual function that accompanies age come problems that are specific to each gender. In women, the most common of these is insufficient vaginal lubrication and an inability to achieve orgasm. In men, erectile dysfunction and health problems come to the forefront.

Age and Sexual Response in Women

Women differ from men in that the decline in sexual responsiveness with aging is quite gradual. The biggest change typically occurs with menopause. As women reach this milestone, hormonal production diminishes and may lead to lubrication deficiency, less genital sensitivity and, for some, a decreased sense of well-being. Many women simply no longer know what to expect when they get sexually aroused. If you anticipate and accept this, menopause does not have to mean the end of a satisfying sex life. In fact, many women report an increased enjoyment of sex because they are no longer worried about unwanted pregnancy.

Lubrication — Lubrication is a very sensitive indicator of sexual arousal in most women. We generally think of it as equivalent to erection in men, though there are exceptions. As women age, their ability to produce lubrication may diminish and sex may become uncomfortable.

Ultimately lubrication is controlled by the autonomic nervous system. Just as your mouth can go dry very quickly in an emergency situation, the same mechanism can cause vaginal lubrication to cease abruptly when a woman perceives something untoward happening — a baby crying, a negative word, a self-conscious thought. With the arrival of menopause, a woman's natural ability to lubricate may diminish. The decline in estrogen levels with menopause can make the vaginal lining thinner and dryer, causing intercourse to be painful for many women. For other women, lack of lubrication will not be an impediment, even after menopause. While it is not clear why, current research suggests there may be a genetic component.

Inability to orgasm — Although many women maintain the capacity to orgasm at near peak levels well into their senior years, most will find the length of time and amount of direct physical stimulation needed to achieve orgasm increases. As women age, the clitoris becomes less engorged with blood during sexual activity and less sensitive, which may cause it to be less stimulated during vaginal intercourse without manual stimulation. For some women, orgasms may be less intense and in some cases uncomfortable. The gradual thinning of vaginal tissue and shortening of the vaginal canal that follows menopause can cause the uterus and the cervix to become smaller. This may result in fewer uterine and vaginal contractions and, in a small number of women, may lead to painful uterine contractions with orgasm.

Age and Sexual Response in Men
Although most will be loath to hear it, there is a strong correlation between age and declining sexual function in men. We can expect that with each decade after middle age, men will have to adjust their expectations of their ability to function sexually.

Most men begin to experience a decrease in their sexual responsiveness, arousability and functioning by age 40. They may find they are less inclined to have sex, that their erections are less frequent or that achieving an orgasm requires more intense stimulation. The good news is that, although these changes are quite noticeable in almost all men by age 60, the pleasure they derive from sex may not be significantly affected. Indeed, recent studies show that most men (unless they have certain health problems) are able to participate in and enjoy sex their entire life span, and many are able to produce viable semen until quite late in life.

Erectile dysfunction — The likelihood of experiencing erectile dysfunction dramatically increases with age. The Massachusetts Male Aging Study found that 52 percent of men age 40 to 70 had some degree of erectile dysfunction. During the late 40s and increasing gradually thereafter, the urgency of sexual interest declines and erection is less frequent and more difficult to sustain, often requiring more intense and continuous direct physical stimulation. Many men begin to experience a periodic inability to achieve erection and will find that the quality of erections is diminished. Erections may not be as hard, ejaculation is less forceful and may not occur with every sexual encounter, and the refractory time between erections is lengthened.

For men with health problems, erectile problems are often compounded. Medical conditions, such as high blood pressure, high cholesterol and diabetes, and the drugs used to treat them, can exacerbate erectile difficulties by blocking blood flow into the penis. Other culprits include anxiety, depression and stress, as well as nerve trauma resulting from spinal cord injury, multiple sclerosis and stroke, prostate or colon diseases.

Regardless of the cause of erectile difficulty, there is always a psychological effect on the male. Men who experience an inability to achieve or sustain an erection on several occasions may be so anxious about inadequacy that they avoid sexual situations and sexual arousal.

Physical health — Physical health issues and aging seem to have a greater impact on men than women when it comes to sexual function. We can only hypothesize why, but it could be related to the fact that men are often hesitant to discuss sexual problems with their clinicians and tend to consult family physicians for health-related problems less frequently than do women. Consequently, men receive fewer medical services, less health information and are less likely to receive advice about how changes in behavior can improve health.

Use it or (Almost) Lose it

Age is not the only factor to consider when it comes to the longevity of your sex life. While the process of aging can dampen sexual functioning, the frequency with which you engage in sexual activity may be a better predictor. A 'use-it-or-lose-it' phenomenon exists for both genders. Less sexual activity tends to contribute to decreased interest and a diminished sexual response. It may also contribute to a decline in the overall sense of well-being. Many couples, particularly those that have been together for a very long time, adjust to relatively low sexual activity in the relationship or even absence of sexual activity, depending more on the companionship of their relationship. Others make adjustments to their sex life and stay sexually active into their 80s and beyond.

STRATEGIES FOR LIFELONG SEX

Aging and the physical changes that go along with it are an inevitable part of life. But it need not be a negative part. Think of the aging process as an opportunity to give your sex life an overhaul and experiment with new techniques, devices and positions.

Imagination

The brain is our most important sexual organ. And it can work for or against you. If you are feeling overwhelmed by pressure at work, are worried about the future of your children or are depressed by your financial circumstances, your interest in sex will likely be low. If, on other hand, you fantasize during the day about the evening ahead with your partner, you're much more likely to engage in intimate activities. A study that examined easily orgasmic women found that fantasy plays a major role in sexual desire. The defining feature of these women was that they were using their brain during the day to conjure erotic images, setting the stage for subsequent sex play with their partner. In effect they had a jump start on the evening ahead. Their engines were running and not in deep freeze mode.

One of the ways you foster sexual energy is by making sure your relationship has a good erotic tone. Erotic tone refers to the special way two people communicate when they choose to share their bodies intimately and it is something that needs to be heeded and honoured. There are a variety of ways to cultivate erotic tone, a good sex life being first and foremost. But it can also be more subtle than that — sexy talk, a certain look or an intimate touch as you pass your partner.

Use a Lubricant

Sex that is uncomfortable quickly becomes undesirable. To counter the effects of menopause, use a personal lubricant. Experiment with a few different brands to find the one best for you. A lubricant can be applied to either partner or, for the most lubrication, to both. Water-based products are preferable to petroleum-based ones. Water-based lubricants that are slightly acidic inhibit the growth of certain harmful microorganisms, such as yeast. Petroleum-based products can adhere to the vaginal walls, providing a place for harmful organisms to multiply, and also damage latex condoms and diaphragms, rendering them ineffective for safe sex.

Make Love in the Morning
If fatigue is getting in the way of your sex life, try making love in the morning. Older men are more likely to have a firm erection in the morning and will function better sexually after a good night's sleep.

Communicate
To deal with dust and debris that builds up on your floors, you vacuum. But how often do you 'vacuum' your relationship? Clear and positive communication with your partner about what you want and what you do not want is arguably the most important part of a healthy sexual relationship. Without open communication, misunderstandings can occur that may lead to the dreaded 'R' condition: Resentment. As we discussed earlier, resentment kills desire. I recommend that all my patients 'vacuum' their relationship at least once a week, usually by appointment.

Limit Alcohol and Tobacco Use
A glass of wine can put you in the mood for intimacy, but too much will put you to sleep. Smoking and excess alcohol are strongly linked to erectile dysfunction in men. Because the likelihood of experiencing erectile dysfunction

increases with age, be sure to avoid alcohol before love making.

Set the Mood

Libido is a delicate flower and requires nurturing. You can't simply wait around to feel sexy. You need to generate desire by setting the mood for sexual arousal. Try sharing a romantic dinner, taking a shower or bath together or exchanging massages. Watch an erotic video or read erotic literature together in bed. Activities like these often naturally lead to sexual relations.

Try a New Position

With age, some people may find that the sexual positions they used when they were younger are no longer comfortable. Try new sexual positions. One effective way for many older adults to have sex is 'on the side'. In this position, the man and woman both lie on their sides with the man 'spooning' the woman. It may take a little practice to get used to, but this position is effective because it allows vaginal intercourse without putting major stress on any joints or necessitating one partner to put his or her weight on the other.

Explore and Discover

For some men and women, vaginal intercourse becomes less probable or even impossible as they age. By no means, however, does this have to be the end of their sex lives. While our society may emphasize vaginal intercourse, there is a vast array of fulfilling sexual acts that go beyond inserting a penis into a vagina. Mutual masturbation, oral sex, shared fantasy, cuddling and kissing can be healthy and fulfilling forms of sexual expression, with or without vaginal intercourse. Or try taking turns giving and receiving sexual pleasure.

Increase Stimulation

Increased genital stimulation can lead to an increase in sexual fulfillment for both men and women. Focus on the buildup, with ample foreplay including non-genital and genital touch prior to penetration. If fatigue is getting in the way, a woman may find a vibrator will give the extra stimulation needed, without wearing out her partner. But be warned; once you start using a vibrator your nervous system can get used to this powerful stimulation (habituation) and you will likely not be able to achieve orgasm without it.

Memory

Dr. Gordon Winocur, PhD

Baycrest Hospital

Henry, an entrepreneur in the technology field, devoted his life to building his small business into a large corporation. Burnt out from years of working long hours, he retired at age 47, determined to break from his career and start enjoying his life. Over the next ten years he half-heartedly pursued a variety of leisure interests and made the odd business deal. But without the high pressure stakes of the corporate world he felt directionless and unchallenged. And it was beginning to show in his day-to-day life. Where he once managed a team of 30 employees, he now had difficultly remembering phone numbers and the dates of important appointments. The more anxious he became about it the worse his memory seemed to get.

More than any other aspect of aging, declining mental faculties seem to be the most difficult to accept. We lose our hair, cannot run as fast, our eyesight starts to fail — we expect these types of changes as we get older and come to terms with them. It follows that we should expect our memory and other aspects of cognitive function to decline as well. But for one reason or another, the expectations we have about our cognitive abilities remain high. Aging of the mind is particularly difficult to deal with.

As we've seen in the previous chapters, aging is a complicated process that is influenced by various biological and non-biological factors. The same holds true in the cognitive domain. Lifestyle and diet have a tremendous impact on brain function. It is well established that obesity, for instance, contributes to cognitive decline and that health conditions like diabetes and high blood pressure, and the medications used to treat them, can impair certain mental processes.

With advancing age, physical changes also take place in the brain. Throughout adulthood, there is a gradual reduction in the weight and volume of the brain, particularly in the hippocampus and the frontal lobes, two structures involved in memory. We can expect these areas of the brain to shrink by about two percent per decade. Connections between neurons, the brain's nerve cells, also shrink in size. Some of the connections may be lost, and new connections may not be made as readily. It is likely that these physical changes account for at least some of the noticeable age-related cognitive changes, though the exact links have not yet been discovered.

Together these factors gradually take their toll on mental ability. One of the first things we notice as we age is a change in memory function or capacity. Our ability to remember specific events, information and experiences is typically the first to go. We may forget to make a deposit at the bank or to return a phone call. We may forget where we left our sun glasses or car keys. Phone numbers may become more difficult to memorize and recall.

By themselves, these types of lapses in memory are easily manageable and do not significantly affect our ability to do things. We can develop strategies to compensate — whether it is writing down important reminders or tying string around a finger. The emotional stress of recognizing these changes, however, can exacerbate the problem. As people become aware of increased absent mindedness, they sometimes get upset by it. They become anxious, even depressed, about declining mental faculties, even though what they are experiencing is perfectly normal. This sets in motion a vicious cycle that makes memory decline, and anxiety about it, progressively worse.

Thankfully, this need not be the case. In fact, we have a certain amount of control over the biological changes of the aging process. Although our bodies are programmed to start to decline as we get older, the specific age at which this process begins is not fixed. There is a window of 20 years or more, depending on several factors, including the individual's lifestyle, before these critical changes take place. By understanding the cognitive changes that occur with age and the various factors that exacerbate cognitive decline, we may be able to slow the process.

AGING AND THE BRAIN

Most studies show that, in general, cognitive abilities are at their peak when people are in their 20s and 30s and, for the most part, remain relatively stable until the 50s or early 60s. After this point these abilities begin to decline, but to varying degrees. In fact, the effects of cognitive changes are sometimes not noticed until the 70s and beyond. It is important to keep these numbers in mind when considering the changes in brain activity and cognitive function discussed below.

Cognitive ability is measured by a number of different skills: intelligence, attention, processing speed and memory; all of which are affected to varying degrees by the aging process.

Fluid and Crystallized Intelligence

Intelligence falls into two categories: namely fluid and crystallized.

Fluid intelligence is an expression of the information processing system. It refers to our ability to deal with situations as they arise. It allows us to perform strategic cognitive functions — to organize, to reason, to solve problems, to make decisions — and includes the speed with which information can be analyzed, as well as attention and memory capacity.

Crystallized intelligence is related to general knowledge. It refers to our ability to manipulate ideas, information and vocabulary accumulated in our experiences over a life span. It also encompasses our ability to apply learned skills and knowledge in order to solve problems.

Many studies have shown that fluid intelligence is more likely to decline with age. Older adults may find it more difficult to learn to play poker or to learn how to use a computer; tasks that require fluid intelligence. This is partly because fluid intelligence depends to a large extent on our use of the frontal lobes, an area of the brain that is one of the first to show structural changes as we get older. On the other hand, crystallized intelligence, which appears to be more widely distributed throughout the brain, may in fact continue to improve with age. Many people continue to gain expertise and skills in particular areas throughout life. A good cook is always a good cook and may add to his or her repertoire of culinary skills at any time in life.

Attention

Attention is the ability to focus on certain bits of information and to decide whether, and how much further, to process it. This skill is necessary for the initial assimilation of information. At any age it is only possible to pay attention to a limited amount of information at one time. In older age, this ability may become more restricted.

Some researchers have found that older adults have difficulty distinguishing between information that is relevant and information that is irrelevant to a particular task, and are susceptible to becoming distracted. This may slow down the speed of performing a mental task and may compromise accuracy.

Processing Speed

From the late 20s on, mental processing and reaction time become slower, albeit imperceptibly at first. In general, by the time most people are 60 or older, they will generally take longer to perform mental tasks than younger people. Older people may take longer to calculate the tip and change on a restaurant bill, or have a hard time keeping a running total on their groceries as they shop. On a positive note, this does not appear to be an indication of declining mental function, but rather a slowing of mental processing. On intelligence tests with liberal time limits, older adults often perform just as well as younger people; it simply takes them longer.

Memory

We tend to overestimate the extent to which we lose memory function as we get older. Memory is not a unitary process. There are many kinds of memory, each with its own operating principles and purpose. While it is true that there is memory decline with age and that memory loss is an early indication of age-related cognitive change, some types of memory are extremely resistant to the aging process.

Semantic memory — Semantic memory represents the everyday facts and experiences we gain over a lifetime, and reflects our overall general knowledge. In most cases we do not usually remember the circumstances under which we learned the information in semantic memory. For instance, everybody knows that if you have a headache you take an aspirin or that when you want to buy tools you go to the hardware store, but you probably do not remember when and where you learned this information. Because semantic memory is related to experience, it remains stable or even improves as we grow older.

Prospective memory — Prospective memory gives you the ability to remember to do something in the future, such as return a book to the library or show up for your next doctor's appointment. Prospective memory can be enhanced with the use of aids or cues, such as 'to do' lists, appointment books and daytimers. Some studies show that prospective memory declines with age while other studies do not. It seems to depend on the specific type of prospective memory task. Well-practiced routines tend to be recalled better, while remembering to perform new tasks requires more effort and attention. Putting things in writing helps prospective memory tremendously. When older adults are allowed to write reminders down or use cues, they do just as well as younger adults on prospective memory tests.

Immediate memory — Imagine going through life not being able to remember what you just said and you will have an idea of what it would be like to lose your immediate memory. Immediate or short-term memory gives you the ability to remember small amounts of information for short periods of time, such as dialing a phone number you've just been told or solving an equation in your head. This ability is crucial for making sense of the world around you. It enables you to follow a book and to have a normal, meaningful conversation. Unlike other types of memory, information in the immediate memory fades quickly, usually after a few seconds. There is a limit to how much can be stored in immediate memory. At any age people can usually store five to seven pieces of information. Happily, this type of memory resists the effects of aging.

Episodic memory — If you are always forgetting where you put your car keys or cannot recall what you had for breakfast, it is most likely a failure of episodic memory. This type of memory is context-dependent and refers to the ability to recall experiences or events that occurred at a particular time and place. Episodic memory is vulnerable to the aging process, especially when subject to longer delays between the event itself and the moment of attempted recall. It is widely held that this is due to a reduced ability to transfer information from immediate or short-term memory to long-term memory. While we tend to fret the most about losing long-term, episodic memory, growing evidence suggests that we may be able to compensate for this by developing appropriate memory strategies.

Remote memory — Remote memory deals with the ability to remember things that happened years ago — attending an aunt's wedding as a child or participating in a grade school play. Remote memory is difficult to study because it is hard to validate whether old personal memories are accurate or not. Older people can often clearly remember an emotional event from years past and re-tell the story, but it is unclear whether it is remote memory or the telling of the story over and over that enables them to remember the details. Remote semantic memories do not appear to be affected by age, while remote episodic memories are not remembered well. You may recall the way you felt on your wedding day and the general highlights of the day, but not all the guests that attended or the time of the ceremony.

COGNITIVE DISORDERS

There is evidence to suggest that changes in the brain begin much sooner than previously thought. With recent advances in neuroimaging techniques and other methods of detection, scientists are identifying very early changes in the brain that seem to be long-term predictors of mental ability down the road. This information enables researchers and doctors to track cognitive function much more easily, but is not necessarily an expression of malfunction early in life. It is simply the very early beginnings of a natural process that will take decades to unfold.

Dementia, in comparison, refers to deterioration of mental functions — memory, language and reasoning — that is caused by disease in the brain. As the disease progresses from mild to severe, dementia interferes with the ability to function independently in everyday life. Dementia is not part of normal aging. Only 7.8 percent of the population over 65 has dementia. That number rises to 37 percent in people over 85 years of age.

Dementia is classified as either cortical (outer brain) or sub-cortical (inner brain), depending on the area of the brain affected. Cortical dementia causes problems in memory, thinking and language, as is seen with Alzheimer's Disease. Sub-cortical dementia affects parts of the brain below the cortex and is characterized by slowing, difficulty in retrieving information from memory and altered mood. Parkinson's Disease and Multiple Sclerosis are conditions that can lead to sub-cortical dementia.

The causes of dementia are not well understood, but there are a number of risk factors associated with the disease. Apart from age, genetics and lifestyle appear to be significant predictors of dementia. For instance, smoking, eating an unbalanced diet and lack of exercise are associated with an increased risk of dementia, as are head injuries and exposure to toxins, like asbestos. The more risk factors you display, the greater your likelihood of developing dementia.

Genetics is another important factor. There is a direct link between dementia and certain genes, accounting for approximately five percent of all dementia cases. Other genes indicate susceptibility to dementia. Research shows people who carry the APOE4 allele gene are more likely to develop dementia than people who do not, particularly when other risk factors are present. If you sustain a head injury as a child and carry the APOE4 allele gene, you are more likely to develop dementia later in life than someone who does not carry the gene.

Mild Cognitive Impairment

Mild cognitive impairment refers to loss of cognitive function that is greater than normal, but is not as significant as dementia. Although not debilitating to the extent that a person cannot function anymore, this condition is a fairly reliable sign that dementia is probable and should be taken seriously.

Caused by an increased rate of shrinkage in the hippocampus, mild cognitive impairment can affect many areas of cognition, including language, attention, critical thinking, reading, writing and memory. This condition can be divided into two broad subtypes: amnestic MCI and non-amnestic MCI. Amnestic MCI is the more debilitating of the two. It significantly affects memory and is linked to Alzheimer's.

The exact prevalence of mild cognitive impairment is difficult to determine. Some estimates are as high as 20 percent of the non-demented population over age 65. However, only about a third of those cases are of the amnestic variety. The risk factors for amnestic MCI are the same as for Alzheimer's — family history, lifestyle and age.

Occasional forgetfulness is nothing to worry about. It is normal to forget where you parked your car sometimes or not to remember the name of a former co-worker when you meet unexpectedly at the grocery store. If you are concerned about starting to forget things you typically remember, such as birthdays or your weekly poker game, it could be a symptom of something more serious and you should consult your doctor.

There is no cure for mild cognitive impairment, but there are drugs that can treat the symptoms and may delay the onset of Alzheimer's in people with amnestic MCI, as well as potentially increasing a person's candidacy for new treatments as they become available.

Alzheimer's Disease

Alzheimer's disease is the most common form of dementia, accounting for 50 percent of all cases. It most often occurs in people over 65, but can affect adults as early as 40. One in 13 Canadians over the age of 65 has Alzheimer's Disease or a related dementia. The longer you live, the greater your risk.

Alzheimer's Disease is a progressive, degenerative disease that destroys vital brain cells, causing a breakdown in the signals they send to each other. As Alzheimer's Disease affects each area of the brain, certain functions or abilities are lost. This results in specific symptoms or changes in behaviour. It is important to remember that once an ability is lost, it is very difficult to reacquire.

It is not known what causes Alzheimer's, but there appear to be genetic, environmental and/or viral components to the disease. If Alzheimer's runs in your family it does not necessarily mean you will develop the disease. Genetics play a direct role in only five to ten percent of all cases. Some individuals who exhibit the APOE4 gene on Chromosome 19 are at increased risk for Alzheimer's Disease but, only in combination with other risk factors. There is no cure for

Alzheimer's Disease but, as with mild cognitive impairment, there are medications and other approaches that can manage some of the symptoms in some people.

STRATEGIES

There is not a lot we can do about declining memory capacity as we age. We can however slow the rate of decline by making positive lifestyle choices that keep the mind and body in top form:

Stay Physically Active

Exercise not only makes you feel more energetic and alert, it is also shown to aid in memory retention and information processing and to improve reaction time, mood, concentration and memory span. It also helps to fend off depression.

Numerous studies have linked physical activity with slower mental decline. In a University of California study, researchers measured the brain function of nearly 6,000 women during an eight-year period. Of the women who exercised the most (17 miles per week) only 17 percent showed significant declines in test scores, compared with 24 percent of the women who exercised the least (a half mile per week). Researchers found that for every extra mile walked per week there was a 13 percent less chance of cognitive decline.

The protective effect of exercise is believed to be related to increased circulation. Exercise increases blood flow to all parts of your body, including your brain, and can cause blood vessels to grow, even in middle-aged sedentary individuals. Walking may be particularly effective at increasing blood flow to the brain. Unlike other forms of exercise, walking increases blood circulation without being strenuous, so the extra oxygen and glucose goes to the brain rather than to muscles in the body. This could be why walking can 'clear your head'.

Exercise is also shown to have a beneficial effect on specific cognitive functions and may even help prevent dementia. In a study by the Duke University Medical Center, exercisers showed significant improvements in the higher mental processes of memory and in 'executive functions' that involve planning, organization and the ability to juggle different intellectual tasks at the same time.

Other studies suggest that exercise reduces the risk of dementia. Exercise and health data from nearly 5,000 men and women over 65 years of age, showed that those who exercised were less likely to lose their mental abilities or develop dementia, including Alzheimer's. The more a person exercises, the greater the protective benefits for the brain. A five-year study at Laval University showed that inactive individuals were twice as likely to develop Alzheimer's, compared to those with the highest levels of activity (exercised vigorously at least three times a week). But even light or moderate exercisers significantly cut their risk for Alzheimer's and mental decline.

To get the mind boosting benefits, you must exercise regularly — at least 30 minutes a day, five to seven days a week. Pick an activity you enjoy, such as working in your garden or walking your dog. If you engage in high impact sports, take precautions to protect your head. Head trauma can increase your risk of developing Alzheimer's. Wear a helmet when riding your bike, skiing or engaging in any high-speed or potentially dangerous sport.

Eat a Balanced Diet

There really is such a thing as brain food. A diet high in antioxidant-rich fruits and vegetables may protect against cognitive decline. Researchers at Tufts University showed that including blueberries, strawberries and spinach in rats' diets reduced, or even reversed, some age-related deficits in short-term memory and motor function.

Conversely, diets high in fat and too high or too low in cholesterol accelerate cognitive decline. A study of over 800 people age 65 and older by the Rush Institute for Healthy Aging found that subjects with the highest intake of saturated or trans fats had more than twice the risk of Alzheimer's Disease compared with people who had the lowest intake of such fats. High intake of unsaturated, unhydrogenated fats seemed to offer a slight protection against Alzheimer's.

Food quantity and frequency of meals can also affect your brain as you age. Researchers at the National Institute on Aging have recently shown that mice fed a calorie-restricted diet or forced to fast every other day are more resistant to degeneration and death of nerve cells and better able to grow new nerve cells. This makes them more resistant to age-related neurodegenerative diseases like Alzheimer's.

Toast to Moderation

Moderate alcohol consumption seems to be protective against dementia. A study of over 700 older adults published in the *Journal of the American Medical Association* showed that participants who consumed between one and six drinks per week were 50 percent less likely than non-drinkers to develop dementia. However, heavy alcohol consumption

(14 or more drinks per week) has the opposite effect. People who drink heavily for years can experience permanent brain damage due to the effects of the alcohol and poor nutrition, and are at increased risk of developing memory problems and dementia.

Keep Your Mind Active

Intellectual pursuits help with memory retention and assist in preventing cognitive disorders. Among other findings, an ongoing study of nuns by the University of Kentucky showed that writing style is an early predictor of Alzheimer's or brain dementia. Researchers found that nuns who were not very expressive in youth showed evidence of very early brain decline, while those who wrote in a rich style and conveyed a great deal of personal information in an interesting way were protected to a much greater extent.

If you continue to challenge yourself, your brain will literally continue to grow. An active brain produces new connections between nerve cells, helping it store and retrieve information more easily. Physical activity is one way to keep your mind fit, but similar evidence is emerging in other areas as well. Learning new skills and taking part in activities that require you to think improves mental agility. Read a book, do a crossword puzzle or attend a lecture. Start a new hobby or learn a foreign language.

Stay Socially Involved and Engaged

With retirement just around the corner, make plans to stay involved. People who have an active social life are able to retain cognitive function significantly better than people who have limited social contacts. They have also been found to live longer, to have better health and to be less depressed. These effects are likely the result of the stimulating and stress-reducing effects of being socially involved.

Social engagement may also be protective against dementia. The Honolulu-Asia Aging Study followed 2,513 elderly Japanese-American men from 1965 and measured levels of social engagement at mid-life and late-life. Researchers found that a low level of mid-life social activity on its own was not associated with an increased risk of dementia. However, any decline in social activity from mid-life into late-life did seem to raise the risk of dementia, as did poor social engagement in late-life.

If you have been a community worker or a pharmacist, for example, plan to stay involved on some level — work part-time or volunteer.

Use Memory Aids

At any age, you are going to forget things. But the older you get the more things you are likely to forget. Make lists, use a daytimer or an electronic diary. Spend a little time each day organizing your tasks for the day, week or month and you will be much less likely to forget an important appointment or meeting. If you find writing bothersome, keep a small tape recorder to capture important appointments or conversations.

If you are interrupted in the middle of a task or something you are reading, take a moment to jot down where you are and the main points of your task. This will help jog your memory once you return to the task.

Mnemonics are also helpful memory-jogging tricks. Use songs, associative rhymes or names to help you retrieve words that are 'on the tip of your tongue'.

How we approach tasks has a dramatic impact on memory. A recent trial conducted by Baycrest Hospital showed that compartmentalizing tasks — breaking complex tasks down into smaller subgoals — in a carefully programmed way makes it much easer to attend to the task at hand without being distracted.

Stay Positive

There is a very important relationship between psychological and social factors and biological changes as far as memory loss and cognitive function are concerned. Research shows that people with high psycho-social function — who are able to stay optimistic and feel in control of their lives — have much higher cognitive function on tests of learning and memory than people who have low self-esteem and do not feel in control of their lives.

In fact, attitude may be the best predictor of how you'll fare, according to a three-year study funded by the National Institute on Aging. In the study, older adults who read a fictional but very negative article on memory and aging performed significantly worse on subsequent memory tests than those who read an equally fictional but positive article on the subject. It goes to show that if exposed enough to a stereotype, we begin to believe it.

Consider Supplements

Certain dietary supplements have been associated with improved cognitive function.

Ginkgo biloba is the world's oldest living species of tree and is often recommended for its effect on memory and cognitive function. Studies suggest that it may enhance cognitive performance in healthy older adults and in people with age-related cognitive decline and Alzheimer's disease. However, strong evidence is lacking.

Those who believe there are medical benefits of ginkgo biloba extract attribute them primarily to two groups of active constituents: the ginkgo flavone glycosides and the terpene lactones. Most clinical trials have used divided doses of 120 and 240 mg of ginkgo biloba (standardized to contain six percent terpene lactones and 24 percent flavone glycosides) per day. Ginkgo biloba may need to be taken for eight to 12 weeks before cognitive improvement is noticed.

Antioxidants are another popular choice. Numerous studies suggest that antioxidants may improve cognitive function and prevent age-related dementia by preventing and repairing free-radical damage in the brain.

Your first line of defence should be eating plenty of antioxidant-rich fruits and vegetables, such as blueberries, bilberries and spinach, but there is evidence that antioxidant supplements have protective effects as well. Vitamin E is particularly thought to improve cognitive function and stall cognitive decline. It is believed that its status as a fat-soluble antioxidant makes it well absorbed by the brain, the body's fattiest organ. Other antioxidant superstars include Vitamin A and C — which, when combined with Vitamin E, may prevent Alzheimer's and vascular dementia — Coenzyme Q10 — which may improve cognitive function — and Grapeseed Extract — for its strong free-radical scavenging properties. Conversely, deficiencies in certain antioxidants may exacerbate cognitive decline. It has been suggested that dementia may occur in those with deficiencies of vitamin B12, as well as deficiencies of the other B vitamins.

Stop Smoking

Memory loss is just one of the many health problems that come from smoking. According to a study by the National Institute on Aging, elderly smokers experience age-related mental decline at five times the rate of their non-smoking counterparts. Among former smokers, the rate of decline is twice that of non-smokers. An earlier study at University College London had similar findings. Studying 2,000 adults, researchers gave participants memory, concentration and visual speed tests at age 43 and again at 53. Heavy smoking — more than 20 cigarettes a day — was associated with faster declines in verbal memory and visual speed.

Other research has identified smoking as a possible contributor to dementia. Smokers may have twice the risk of getting Alzheimer's Disease as do people who have never smoked.

It's never too late to stop. If you quit smoking now, you can still reduce health-related risks, which include memory loss.

As we age, our ability to remember specific events, experiences and information wanes. We may forget what we watched on the news last night or what we had for breakfast. While these occasional lapses have little impact on our life, we naturally become concerned about declining cognitive function, often exaggerating and exacerbating the rate of decline. If you are experiencing memory loss, discuss your concerns with your doctor. He or she can look at your overall health and perform exams to either reassure you or to determine if further intervention is necessary. If you are concerned about memory loss down the road, implement preventative strategies. Exercise your body and mind, eat a healthy diet and be engaged in life and you'll increase your chances of retaining a sharp memory.

Mind, Body and Soul

By Dr. Elaine Dembe, DC

Chiropractor, Author, Inspirational Speaker

For Barbara, a widowed housewife, life at 52 was not what she expected. Her three children grown and moved out and her husband deceased, she found herself alone at a time when she imagined she would be enjoying winters in Florida and summers at the cottage with her life partner. Every year, instead of taking a trip she found a reason to stay behind. Clinging to her grief and loneliness, Barbara realized her life was on hold. She was wasting away her freedom years.

As we age, we become acutely aware of the ebb and flow of life — the beginnings and the inevitable endings yet to come. The days, weeks, years fly by. The possessions that once seemed so important lose value, and the relationships in our lives become all the more significant. At 50 comes the realization that life is short and must be celebrated everyday.

In the previous chapters we discussed the mechanics of Aging Smart, but that only tells part of the story. Aging Smart is not only about our physical wellness. It involves our whole being; an interconnection of three elements — body, mind and soul. Science shows us that how we feel emotionally has a tremendous impact on our physical health; particularly our immune system. It follows that the final chapter in this book be devoted to cultivating our spiritual and emotional well-being.

In today's fast-forward society it is easy to get caught up in what we have to accomplish and what lies ahead. Often we are so focused on waiting for big things to make us happy that we miss the small, ordinary, everyday things that bring joy and meaning to our lives.

Joy is central to a meaningful existence and, once you become aware of the possibilities, it is everywhere to be had. Joy is what moves you deeply, what stirs your soul, what makes your eyes moist, what ignites your heart. Joy is in whatever plucks the strings of passion in your heart; in the very depths of your being. Joy is in the wonder of a child, in the poignancy of life, in the overflowing love for someone. Joy is found in the life cycle — melting snow making way for the tender green shoots of spring. Joy is in gratitude, in the surprise and privilege of waking up in the morning. Joy is in the temporary; in the moments that don't last, the day that is gone before we know it, the life that is over so quickly.

Don't postpone joy. By following a few simple principles you can find joy in the everyday:

Learn to Adapt
Something happens at around 50; you finally begin to make

peace with the body you are given. I no longer sigh with envy while looking at magazines featuring supermodels strutting their tight butts in thong underwear. Now that I am on my third box of birthday candles (there are 24 in a box!), I accept that: a) I'll never be a supermodel and, b) I have spider veins, bunions, a few wrinkles, some brown spots and receding gums. And I'm okay with it.

Like me, many baby boomers are coming to terms with mid-life and aging issues. Let's face it, aging sneaks in the back door while we are living life. At mid-life, we must be aware of two realities: we are not immortal and loss is inevitable. You may have already experienced major losses, such as the death of a parent, the end of a marriage or significant relationship, a job or career termination or a change in physical health. Unfortunately, as we age, we also understand that others age with us, so there are more losses yet to come.

As psychiatrist Dr. Howard Book explains, "We must adapt the way we think, feel and behave to changing situations and circumstances. A component of adapting is acceptance — the ability to acknowledge our strengths and weaknesses and feel good about ourselves nonetheless."

For some, accepting our limitations means changing the way we think about our bodies. We must recognize that we cannot control every aspect of what happens to us. For others, it means changing the way we think about our partner. At mid-life and beyond, the rules change. The initial contract that we agreed upon as a couple acquires addenda. Health changes, career challenges, retirement and the empty-nest syndrome all affect a couple's relationship. You may find your goals, or those of your partner, change at mid-life. Perhaps you want to settle down into a quieter life, or this could be the time you finally start your own business. As you change as individuals, you change what being a couple now means. Together you must adapt or your relationship will suffer. Acceptance doesn't mean we have to like what happens. No one welcomes adversity. But denying it, or wishing it away, is not the answer either. Acceptance is a process — an evolution. You don't just wake up and accept a situation, but over time come to terms with your inability to change it — and then change your attitude instead.

When it comes to the loss of someone you love, acceptance is the most difficult path that we must walk. We struggle with the finality, the reality, of what has occurred. No loss is ever completely mourned. We are never finished with the process of acceptance. Even years after we have lost a loved one, like a broken glass that has shattered into millions of tiny fragments, a sliver can pierce us when we least expect it. Remembering a birthday, sharing a memory, celebrating a family tradition without that person, or attending another funeral — all of these and more can open up our sadness as if the loss had just happened. During the busyness of our day we may laugh and carry on with no hint of sorrow on our face. But at night, in a darkened room, alone with our thoughts, tears may fall. Understand that these emotions will revisit us indefinitely. Acceptance involves peeling the sorrowful layers away to a deeper core of healing.

When we learn to accept life just as it is, even with our own unchosen landscape of difficulties, pain and loss, we learn to live fully with the course that life chooses for us. We change the way we relate to suffering by opening up our hearts to love, and miracles happen. Our pain often motivates us to help others, or puts us in touch with inner strengths we did not know existed.

Embrace Resilience

One of the basic tenets of life is that nothing ever remains the same. Life is constantly evolving and we must adapt to it. We all know individuals who thrive in the face of change and others who rigidly resist.

The difference lies in how we choose to react to change. Those who flourish have developed inner resources to adjust to changing circumstances. They demonstrate optimism and hope, high self-esteem, confidence and resilience — no matter what happens — to cope with the stresses of life. They accept that crisis and change are normal companions throughout life. Do not be afraid to shift, adjust or alter your perception.

This means approaching expectations without attachment. When we invest too heavily in any one outcome (the eggs-in-one-basket principle) we set ourselves up for disappointment. We must learn to renegotiate life with every challenge. When we do this, we learn to trust the process and we are more accepting when we don't get what we wanted or expected. We are more philosophical, understanding that life is unfolding as it should.

Every disappointment is an opportunity for us to re-evaluate, to get a reading on how well we have assessed the reality of a situation. If we see it in an optimistic way, disappointment can be a friend, an ally in our search for a joyful life. It can motivate us to learn from our negative and painful experiences.

Live in the Moment

We've all had the experience of someone not 'being in the room' with us. Can you remember talking with someone at a cocktail party who was more interested in checking out other guests than in your conversation? Being in the room is part of a larger concept — being in the world. Many individuals sleepwalk through life. On automatic pilot, they only go through the motions of living. They may see the big picture but fail to focus on the details. They drive home from work but fail to notice the fiery sunset reflecting brilliant gold off office windows. Or they may eat dinner oblivious to the colour and tastes of the food and garnishes, or to the bouquet of spring flowers that adorns the table.

These small, ordinary, everyday moments keep our lives joyful and fresh. Life is then lived like an exclamation mark! To live fully each day we must pay attention and be mindful of everything. When you live this way, you anchor yourself in the present. This present-moment awareness is often called mindfulness. Derived from Zen Buddhism, it is a form of meditation in which you focus your attention on what you are experiencing from moment to moment. You don't think about what you are going to do next or what happened yesterday.

We can all learn to pay attention, to be more present and mindful of everyday life. Start with just one experience, and then move on to another:

- Take a shower and be in touch with your body, the sounds of the water, the smell of the soap, the sensations on your skin
- Eat an orange. Be mindful of the taste, the smells, the

juice, the chewing and swallowing mechanism
- When you are stopped at a red light, see this as an opportunity to take a full breath and relax
- When working out at the gym, don't watch television or use an iPod. Be with your breath and with whatever your body is experiencing. Pay attention to how your muscles feel
- When having a massage, pay attention to each stroke and to your breathing
- When you are outside, notice something pleasant each day, such as clouds, flowers or leaves gently moving in the wind

Contemplating these small pleasures brings joy to our daily lives. We'll miss the little gems that occur every day if we wait to be joyful only about the big things in life, such as meeting the right person, or achieving financial security. We'll miss the best moments if we're too caught up in keeping pace with today's frantic world. In the over-all scheme of things, each moment is like a heartbeat; just as one heartbeat multiplied millions of times creates the continuous flow of life, these small joys multiply to give continuous life to our days.

Don't postpone joy. It is there for you in small ways every single day. A smile, a hug, a kind word, a flower, a book or a song may make all the difference. All you have to do is open your eyes and seize the moment.

Unburden Your Life and Self

As we age, we become more aware of the passage of time. When you find yourself praying for voice mail because a 'live' conversation takes too long, learning to say no is a necessity. No is a choice; the challenge is to stay focused and make choices that align with your goals.

For many of us, turning 50 represents a growing awareness of our need for physical, emotional and spiritual well-being. In the strainer of life we have sifted out the lumps that clog up our karma — people who drain our energy, and obligations that no longer make sense. At a certain point you have to decide to please yourself. Although it is not always easy to do, it gets easier with age and at 50 you still have time to get it right. Start small, by making choices that simplify your life:

Ear-rings — Your cellphone is not an appendage hanging from your ear, so don't treat it like one. Keep it out of restaurants and theatres. Unplug, or switch off your telephone when you do not want to be disturbed.

De-clutter — Clutter is an energy drain. Think of the time it takes just to find things, not to mention the effort expended deciding where to put everything. As your life evolves, you will find meaning in relationships and activities, not things. Letting go of the clutter in your life can be a liberating experience. Start with one small chore, like sorting out your shoes and boots. Give those pointy-toed four-inch heels to the nearest teenager. Next, tackle your kitchen junk drawer ... and so on.

RSVP (reject s'il vous plaît) — Every time you receive an invitation, ask yourself, "Do I really want to go? How important is this relationship to me? Is there something else I'd rather be doing instead? Am I saying yes out of obligation or will I feel guilty if I say no?" Sometimes, even when we don't want to go, we need to do the right thing to support and help others, but otherwise we have to learn to say no, especially when we have so little valuable time on our hands.

Find your dream team — How much is your time and energy worth? Hire people who can do it better, faster and more easily than you. On occasion, hiring a cleaning lady, tailor or gardener can greatly reduce your stress level. A session with a personal trainer can keep you motivated and fit.

Me-time — Sitting in the backyard studying cloud formations is not a waste of time. Contemplation, meditation and taking a slow walk are all healing ways to keep us peaceful and in the moment.

No regrets — We are all human and make mistakes. Often it is not the choice that is problematic but the way we feel about a choice we made. If you are torturing yourself with regret, why not try to change your future? If you truly want to, you can make a concerted effort to find your passion, change your career, make health a priority or quit smoking. As for the most difficult relationship regrets, stop looking back over your shoulder. Forgive yourself and others, and ultimately accept what is.

Find Balance

Balance is a concept that is as difficult to achieve as it is to define. In work and life, it is like chasing the impossible dream. To me, balance is about the choices we make in life — the things we make priorities and that give us meaning.

There are often huge gaps between what people say they think is important and how they actually spend their time.

Part of the problem is the way we think of balance. People often treat balance as if it is something tangible. A better way to define it is as an outcome; balance is achieved when the things we do result in achievement and joy. You may not always be able to spend as much time on one area of your life as you would like, but if you can find joy in most aspects of it — your work, your family, your relationships — you will have balance, or something close to it.

Remember What was

In our forward-looking society, we spend much time planning, scheming and daydreaming about the future. When we spend too much time looking forward, we neglect the richness of our own personal history. Life then becomes meaningless, fragmented and hollow. All of us have experienced thousands of happy moments in our lives. Too often they remain buried under the rubble of the everyday worries and problems that take up space in our heads.

Happy memories counterbalance the negative in our lives and remind us to be thankful. They also benefit our immune system. Happy feelings increase the number of disease-fighting natural killer cells — the body's police force — which may help to explain why optimists are often healthier and live longer than pessimists.

One way to reconnect with happy memories is by recalling the rituals and traditions in our lives. Rituals connect us with our past and provide continuity in the present. Ceremonies and traditions link us to future generations. Rituals are not mindless routines, as they give our life meaning, shape and a sense of harmony and rhythm. Rituals also give families a feeling of cohesion.

Rituals need not be profound to be significant. Birthdays, holidays, graduation and reunions are all celebrations of everyday life. Rites of passage; those things that we do for the first time, and have always been celebrated by humanity also need to be acknowledged. Even ordinary activities — like riding a bike, driving a car, leaving home for university or a first job — can be transformed into significant events when they are honoured with love and a sense of wonder.

It is not enough to remember our rituals and traditions; we must keep them alive and pass them on to future generations. Get your family together and revive the traditions that may have been lost or forgotten, or start new ones. Dig out, or re-create, some recipes that you loved as a kid.

Find the Child Within

Play, it turns out, is not a waste of time. Mounting evidence suggests that play reduces stress levels, restores optimism, refreshes spirits and stimulates creativity. Those who play regularly may even live longer and be happier.

Part of the 'play prescription' is laughter. Scientific studies confirm that laughter is not only good for our emotional health, but it also accelerates healing by stimulating the immune system. Humour also helps us to cope with whatever challenges we are facing in life, and acts as a catalyst to allow us to move through loss or grief.

What counts as play to you will depend on your interests. You may count rock climbing or chess as play time, or enjoy a rousing game of scrabble. For others the exuberance and boundless energy of children or the thumping tail of a favourite pet fill the play time void. If there is not enough play in your life, think about returning to the things that you loved learning as a child or a teenager. Tapping into the activities that we used to love can be fun, playful and healing the second time around.

Live for the Adventure

Though courage is a part of our everyday lives, few people admit to being courageous, believing it to be associated mainly with exceptional risks and heroic deeds. It takes courage to express our true feelings, to believe in our ideas or to face what we fear. It is an act of courage to take risks, to say no, to make changes in our lives — big and small. When faced with pain and adversity, just getting out of bed in the morning may be courageous. We also demonstrate the courage to persevere after the loss of loved ones.

Courage teaches us to grow, learn and stretch beyond our boundaries as we deal with life's challenges. At mid-life many people finally find the courage to 'do it now', whether 'it' means beginning a new career, simplifying one's living space, pursuing creative interests or changing one's marital status. Even for those who feel they have to consider others first — children, parents, spouse — mid-life can still unleash a tremendous sense of freedom to pursue what lies in the heart.

It is normal to feel fear when heading down a new path, but the alternative is even more terrifying. Avoiding risk is like going through life unplugged. Your screen is blank. There is no history to be savoured or saved. We learn the most about ourselves when we leave the safety of a well-worn route. Acknowledge your sweaty palms. Accept that you may feel ambivalent as a new opportunity, challenge or change presents itself. Are there any 'boogeymen' blocking your trail? Go around them. Or move sideways for as long as you need to, then climb higher or dig deeper. Just move. Staying still is just as bad as moving backwards.

Give and you Shall Receive

The most meaningful gifts come from the heart. Giving is about the small joys that we receive in our lives and the people who give them to us. There are gifts of compassion — volunteering to help others in need — and gifts of friendship.

Compassion, or humanness, at the most basic level involves caring about others. Whether it is helping someone who appears lost, picking up a discarded pop can on the sidewalk or just saying thanks to the person who pumps your gas, humanness requires that you think of others. The Golden Rule — do unto others as you would have them do unto you — is the most thoughtful rule to live by. When you value and cherish the people who give to you, then you will gladly bring joy into other people's lives with the same generosity of spirit.

Gifts of friendship, the magic connection between two people, are some of the most profound. Even with some neglect, there are usually enough sparks to keep the embers of a relationship warm. An e-mail or phone call may be enough to stoke it regularly and a face-to-face get together can restore the crackling fires. Deep friendships have no boundaries. These are the friends who mourn with you, fly out for your wedding or make the best dates when you are alone on New Year's. Cheerleaders, chauffeurs and surrogate parents — best friends are there for each other. They are the joy in everyday life!

Giving not only makes you feel good, but it may also help you live longer. Anyone who has ladled soup for the homeless or sorted donated toys for needy children at Christmas returns home with a warm heart and a boost to their immune system. According to scientific studies, there is a physiological response called 'helper's high' that releases brain chemicals known to decrease the stress response. This feel-good factor counteracts negative stress, which is a major factor in disease.

Celebrate Life

Think about your life story so far. Do you value, appreciate and celebrate everything you've learned? If I asked you to tell me your best life stories, would you eliminate the painful ones? We need to understand that all of our experiences are life's best stories.

Look around and you will see that everyone's life has its measure of joy and difficulties. Happy, optimistic people appreciate and accept that fact. Joy and happiness are part of our being, just like breathing. No one has to remind us to breathe; joy should be automatic as well.

As you continue on your journey through life, live with the knowledge that each day is a gift — a day for you to cherish. Suck the juices out of life! Live like an exclamation mark! Every day offers a thousand moments to learn, play, laugh, love, give or just be. When you live and breathe those moments each day, your life will be overflowing with joy.

Michele Sevier's Supplement Guide

Chapter One: Aging Smart

Supplement recommendations

Multivitamin/mineral formulation

Greens product

Essential fatty acids

Antioxidants

Vitamin A, C, E (natural form) and selenium

Glutathione (reduced form)

CoQ10

Alpha lipoic Acid (r-alpha lipoic acid)

Zinc

Flavonoids including anthocyanidins, polyphenols, quercetin

Grape seed extract

Pine bark

Note: Antioxidant supplements are best taken in the form of combination products, as multiple antioxidants appear to work together synergistically far more effectively than a single antioxidant.

Chapter Two: Nutrition
Supplement recommendations
Multivitamin/mineral formulation
Greens product
Essential fatty acids
Whey protein
Soy protein
Probiotics
Digestive enzymes
Anti-inflammatories including ginger, turmeric, bromelain, papain

Chapter Three: Fitness
Supplement recommendations
Multivitamin/mineral formulation
Greens product
Essential fatty acids
Whey protein
Soy protein

Chapter Four: Weight Management
Supplement recommendations
Multivitamin/mineral formulation
Greens product
Essential fatty acids
Protein (Whey or Soy)
Fibre

Chromium
Fat Burner/Thermogenic product
Coleus forskohlii
Gymnema
Citrus aurantium
CLA
Green tea
HCA
White kidney bean
Proteinase inhibitor

Chapter Five: Appearance
Supplement recommendations
Multivitamin/mineral formulation
Greens product
Essential fatty acids
Protein (Whey or Soy)

Antioxidants
Vitamin A, C, E (natural form) and selenium
Glutathione (reduced form)
CoQ10
Alpha lipoic Acid (r-alpha lipoic acid)
Zinc
Flavonoids including anthocyanidins, polyphenols, quercetin
Grape seed extract
Pine bark

Note: Antioxidant supplements are best taken in the form of combination products, as multiple antioxidants appear to work together synergistically far more effectively than a single antioxidant.

Additionally choose topical skin preparations (cleansers, toners, moisturizing creams) that include antioxidant ingredients.

Chapter Six: Stress
Supplement recommendations
Multivitamin/mineral formulation
Greens product
Essential fatty acids
Protein (Whey or Soy)
Relora
Rhodiola
L-Theanine
High potency B vitamins
Holy basil
Schizandra berry
Siberian ginseng

Chapter Seven: Sleep
Supplement recommendations
Multivitamin/mineral formulation
Greens product
Essential fatty acids
Melatonin
Gaba
5-HTP
Magnesium
Valerian

Chapter Eight: Sex
Supplement recommendations
Multivitamin/mineral formulation
Greens product

Supplement Guide

Essential fatty acids
Maca
Ashwagandha
Males — Tribulus, horny goat weed, zinc
Females — Damiana

Chapter Nine: Memory
Supplement recommendations
Multivitamin/mineral formulation
Greens product
Essential fatty acids
Lecithin
Phosphatidylserine
Phosphotidylcholine
Gingko biloba
Taurine
Tyrosine

Chapter Ten: Mind, Body & Soul
Supplement recommendations
Multivitamin/mineral formulation
Greens product
Essential fatty acids
Whey or Soy protein

Michele Sevier is a Doctor of Natural Medicine and independent advisor to Nutrition House Canada. For more information on these and other supplements visit:
www.nutritionhouse.ca

References

Chapter One: Aging Smart

Hoyert, D. L., Heron, M., Murphy, S. L. et al., *Deaths: Final data for 2003*. National Centre for Health Statistics. Health E-Stats. Released January 19, 2006. http://www.cdc.gov/nchs/products/pubs/pubd/hestats/finaldeaths03/finaldeaths03.htm

Rowe, J.W. and Kahn, R.L., *Successful Aging: The MacArthur Foundation Study*. Dell Publishing, New York, 1998.

Bray, T.M., Taylor, C.G., *Tissue Glutathione, Nutrition and Oxidative Stress*. Can J Physiol Pharmacol 1993; 71: 746–751.

Cross, C.E., Traber, M., Eiserich, J., *Micronutrient Antioxidants and Smoking*. Brit Med Bull 1999; 53: 691–704.

Fernandez-Checa, J.C., Kaplowitz, N., Garcia-Ruiz, C., *Mitochondrial Glutathione: Importance and Transport*. Seminars in Liver Dis. 1998; 18: 389–401.

Grossi, S.G., Skrepcinski, F.B., DeCaro, T. et al., *Treatment of Periodontal Disease in Diabetics Reduces Glycated Hemoglobin.* J. Periodont 1997; 68: 713–719.

Jones, D.P., *Glutathione Distribution in Natural Products: Absorption and Tissue Distribution.* Methods Enzymol 1995; 252 3–13.

Jones, D.P., Coates, R.J., Flagg, E.W. et al., *Glutathione in Foods Listed in the National Cancer Institute's Health Habits and History Food Frequency Questionnaire.* Nutr Cancer 1992; 17: 57–75.

Milliman, W.B., Lamson, D.W., Brignall, M.S., *Hepatitis C: A Retrospective Study.* Alternat Med Review 2000; 5: 355–370.

Podmore, I.D., Griffiths, H.R., Herbert, K.E. et al., *Vitamin C Exhibits Pro-oxidant Activities.* Nature 1998; 392: 559.

Rayman, M.P., *The Importance of Selenium to Human Health.* The Lancet 2000; 356: 233–241.

Samiec, P.S., Drews-Botsch, C., Flagg, E.W. et al., *Glutathione in Human Plasma: Decline in Association with Aging, Age-related Macular Degeneration and Diabetes.* Free Radic Biol Med 1998; 15: 699–704.

Steenvoorden, D.P.I., Van Henegouwen, G.M., *The Use of Endogenous Antioxidants to Improve Photoprotection.* J. Photochem Photobiol, B. 41:1–10, 1997.

Chapter Two: Nutrition

Brodb, S.A., *Unregulated inflammation shortens human functional longevity.* Inflammation Res. November 2000; 49 (11): 561–70.

Canadian Cancer Society, *Quick facts on cancer.* http://www.cancer.ca/ccs/internet/standard/0,3182,3172_15306__langId-en,00.html

Statistics Canada, *Causes of Death 2002*. December 6, 2004 Cat. 84-208-XIE. http://www.statcan.ca/english/freepub/ 84-208-XIE/84-208-XIE2004002.htm

American Heart Association, *Menopause and the risk of heart disease and stroke*. http://www.americanheart.org/presenter. jhtml?identifier=4658

Heart and Stroke Foundation. Healthy Living. Healthy Eating. *Legumes for Heart Health*. Dec 17, 2001. http:// ww2.heartandstroke.ca/Page.asp?PageID=33&ArticleID=9 33&Src=living&From=SubCategory

Heart and Stroke Foundation. Healthy Living. Healthy Eating. *What foods are the most useful in preventing cardiovascular disease?* Dec. 17, 2001. http://ww2.heartandstroke.ca/ Page.asp?PageID=33&ArticleID=928&Src=living&From= SubCategory

American Heart Association, *Statistical Fact Sheet: Nutrition and Cardiovascular Disease*. Behavioral Risk Factor Surveillance Study [1990-96], Centers for Disease Control and Prevention/National Center for Health Statistics http://www.americanheart.org/downloadable/heart/111161 2169698FS24NUT5.REVdoc.doc

Invitti, C., *Obesity and low-grade systemic inflammation*. Minerva Endocrinol. September 2002; 27(3): 209–14.

Lindahl, B. et al., *Markers of myocardial damage and inflammation in relation to long-term mortality in unstable coronary artery disease. FRISC Study Group. Fragmin during Instability in Coronary Artery Disease*. New England Journal of Medicine. October 19, 2000; 343(16): 1139–47.

Schanfarber, L., Alive magazine. October 2004; 264: 24.

Conor, W., *Importance of n-3 fatty acids in health ad disease*. American Journal of Clinical Nutrition January 2000; 71: 171S–175.

Koh-Banerjee, P. et al., *Changes in whole-grain, bran and cereal fiber consumption in relation to 8-y weight gain among men.* American Journal of Clinical Nutrition November 2004; 80: 1237–1245.

Simopoulos, A.P., *Omega-3 fatty acids in health and disease and in growth and development.* American Journal of Clinical Nutrition September 1991; 54: 438–463.

Weil, A., *Eating Well for Optimal Health-The Essential Guide to Bringing Health and Pleasure Back to Eating.* Harper Collins, 2001.

Toohey and Kreutle, *Nutritional Physiology: Clinical Applications and Scientific Research.* HealthQuest Publishing, Fort Collins, CO, 1995.

Fletcher, R. H., Fairfield, K. M., *Vitamins for Chronic Disease Prevention in Adults.* JAMA. 2002;287:3127–3129.

Shulman, J., *The Natural Makeover Diet: A 4-Step Program to Looking and Feeling your Best from the Inside Out.* John Wiley & Sons Canada, Ltd. 2005.

von Schacky, C., Angerer, P., Kothny, W. et al., *The effect of dietary omega-3 fatty acids on coronary atherosclerosis. A randomized, double-blind, placebo-controlled trial.* Ann Intern Med 1999;130:554–62.

Mate, J., Castanos, R., Garcia-Samaniego, J., Pajares, J. M., *Does dietary fish oil maintain the remission of Crohn's disease: a case control study.* Gastroenterology 1991;100: A228 [abstract].

Kremer, J. M., Lawrence, D. A., Petrillow, G. F. et al., *Effects of highdose fish oil on rheumatoid arthritis after stopping nonsteroidal antiinflammatory drugs.* Arthritis Rheum 1995;38:1107–14.

Shahar, E., Folsom, A. R., Melnick, S. L. et al., *Dietary n-3 polyunsaturated fatty acids and smoking-related chronic* obstructive pulmonary disease. *Atherosclerosis Risk in Communities Study Investigators*. N Engl J Med, 1994; 331:228–33.

Zhu, Z. R., Mannisto, J. A. S., Pietinene, P. et al., *Fatty acid composition of breast adipose tissue in breast cancer patients and patients with benign breast disease*. Nutr Cancer 1995;24:151–60.

Edwards, R., Peet, M., Shay, J., Horrobin, D., *Omega-3 polyunsaturated fatty acid levels in the diet and in red blood cell membranes of depressed patients*. J Affect Disord 1998;48:149–55.

Smirnov, V. V., Reznik, S. R., V'iunitskaia, V. A. et al., *The current concepts of the mechanisms of the therapeutic-prophylactic action of probiotics from bacteria in the genus bacillus*. Mikrobiolohichnyi Zhurnal, 1993;55:92–112.

Arunachalam, K., Gill, H. S., Chandra, R. K., *Enhancement of natural immune function by dietary consumption of Bifidobacterium lactis* (HN019). Eur J Clin Nutr 2000;54:263–7.

McDonough, F. E., Hitchins, A. D., Wong, N. P. et al., *Modification of sweet acidophilus milk to improve utilization by lactose-intolerant persons*. Am J Clin Nutr 1987;45:570–4.

Chapter Three: Fitness

andropause.ca, *About Andropause*. http://www.andropause.ca/en/about/

MayoClinic.com, *Tools for healthier lives. WOMEN'S HEALTH. Perimenopause*.

http://www.mayoclinic.com/health/perimenopause/DS00554/DSECTION=2

Harvard Men's Health Watch, *Exercise and aging: Can you walk away from Father Time?* Harvard Health Publications

December 2005.

Bartholomew, J. B., Morrison, D., and Ciccolo, J. T., *Effects of Acute Exercise on Mood and Well-Being in Patients with Major Depressive Disorder.* Medicine & Science in Sports & Exercise. 37(12):2032-2037, December 2005.

McKenna, J. et al., *Study: Workers more productive after exercise.* 52nd American College of Sports Medicine (ACSM) Annual Meeting in Nashville, Tenn. June 2005.

Fang, J., Wylie-Rosett, J., Cohen, H. W. et al., *Exercise, body mass index, caloric intake, and cardiovascular mortality.* Am J of Prev Med. Nov 2003 Vol 25;4;283–289.

Stewart, K. J., Bacher, A. C., Hees, P. S. et al., *Exercise Effects on Bone Mineral Density: Relationships to Changes in Fitness and Fatness.* American Journal of Preventive Medicine, Vol 28; Issue 5; 453–460, June 2005.

Yaffe, K., Barnes, D., Nevitt, M. et al., *A prospective study of physical activity and cognitive decline in elderly women.* Arch of Intern Med 2001; 161: 1703–1708.

Physical Activity Readiness Questionnaire (PAR-Q). Public Health Agency of Canada. http://www.phac-aspc.gc.ca/pau-uap/fitness/questionnaire.html

Schneider, E., *The Longevity Quotient: Calculate Your Odds of Aging Well-and Take Steps Now to Stay Youthful for Life.* Rodale, 2003.

Chapter Four: Weight Management

Obesity statistics for Canadian Adults. Health Canada. *Canadian Community Health Survey* 2000/2001 http://www.statcan.ca/Daily/English/020508/d020508a.htm

Salinsky, E. and Scott, W., *Obesity in America: A Growing Threat.* National Health Policy Forum Background Paper, July 11, 2003, Washington, DC.

American Public Health Association. *Testimony of the National Alliance for Nutrition and Activity (NANA).* House Appropriations Subcommittee on Labor, Health and Human Services, Education, and Related Agencies, April 30, 2002.

Cleland, R. L., Gross, W. C., Koss, L. D. et al., *Weight Loss Advertising: An Analysis of Current Trends.* Report to the Staff of the Federal Trade Commission, September 2002.

Lean, M.E. et al., *Waist Circumference as a measure for indicating need for weight management.* BMJ 1995; 311:158–161.

Rowe, J.W. and Kahn, R.L., *Successful Aging: The MacArthur Foundation Study.* Dell Publishing, New York, 1998.

Taheri, S., Ling, L., Austin, D. et al., *Short Sleep Duration Is Associated with Reduced Leptin, Elevated Ghrelin, and Increased Body Mass Index.* Public Library of Science online vol. 1 Issue 3, December 2004. http://biology.plos journals.org/perlserv/?request=getdocument&doi=10.1371 /journal.pmed.001062

Dietary Reference Intakes for Energy, Carbohydrate, Fiber, Fat, Fatty Acids, Cholesterol, Protein, and Amino Acids (Macronutrients) National Academy of Sciences, May 2, 2001. http://www.iom.edu/CMS/3788/4576/4340.aspx

Blankson, H., Stakkestad, J.A., Fagertun, H. et al., *Conjugated linoleic acid reduces body fat mass in overweight and obese humans.* J Nutr. December 2000; 130 (12): 2943–8.

Gaullier, J.M., Halse, J., Hoye, K. et al., *Conjugated linoleic acid supplementation for 1 y reduces body fat mass in healthy overweight humans.* Am J Clin Nutr 2004: 79: 1118–25.

MacDonald, H.B., *Conjugated linoleic acid and disease prevention: a review of current knowledge.* Journal of the

Amer-Coll of Nutrition 2000; 19(2): 111S–118S.

Riserus, U., Berlund, L., Vessby, B., *Conjugated linoleic acid (CLA) reduced abdominal adipose tissue in obese middle-aged men with signs of the metabolic syndrome: a randomised controlled trial.* Int J Obes Rekzt Metah Disord, August 2001; 25(8): 1129–35.

Smedman, A., Vessby, B., *Conjugated linoleic acid supplementation in humans-metabolic effects.* Lipids, August 2001; 36(8): 773–81.

Chantre, P., Lairon, D., *Recent findings of green tea extract AR25(Exolise) and its activity for the treatment of obesity.* Phytomedicine 2002; 9:3–8.

Dulloo, A.G., Duret, C., Rohrer, D. et al., *Efficacy of a green tea extract rich in catechin polyphenols and caffeine in increasing 24-h energy expenditure and fat oxidation in humans.* Am J Clin Nutr 1999; 70: 1040–5.

Preuss, H.G., Bagchi, D., Bagchi, M., Rao, C.V.S., Satyan-arayana, S., Dey, D.K., *Efficacy of a Novel, Natural Extract of (-) Hydroxycitric Acid (HCA-SX) and a Combination of HCA-SX, Niacin-Bound Chromium and Gymnema sylvestre Extract in Weight Management in Human Volunteers: A Pilot Study.* Nutrition Research 2004; 24: 45–58.

Preuss, H.G., Bagchi, D., Bagchi, M., Rao, C.V.S. et al., *Effects of a Natural Extract of (-) Hydroxycitric Acid (HCA-SX) and a Combination of HCA-SX plus Niacin-Bound Chromium and Gymnema sylvestre Extract on Weight Loss.* Diabetes, Obesity and Metabolism 2004; 6: 171–180.

Udani, J., Hardy, M., and Madsen, D. C., *Use of Phase 2 Starch Neutralizer(tm)-brand bean extract for weight loss: a randomized controlled trial.* Northridge Hospital Medical Center, UCLA. http://www.phase2info.com/clin_studies/study_starchtrial.asp

Kopelman, P. and Lennard-Jones, J., *Nutrition and patients: a doctor's responsibility*. Clin Med JRCPL 2002;2:391–4

Torkos, S., *Winning at Weight Loss: Proven strategies based on diet, exercise & supplements*. John Wiley & Sons, Canada, 2004.

Chapter Five: Appearance

Rook, A., Wilkinson, D.S. and Ebling, S.J.G. (editors), *The Normal Skin. Textbook of Dermatology* Volume 1 3rd edition 1968; 5–30.

Balan, A.K., Klignman, A.M., *Skin and Aging*. New York: Raven Press, 1989.

Fisher, G. J., Wang, Z., Datta, S.C. et al., *Pathophysiology of Premature Skin Aging Induced by Ultraviolet Light*. New England Journal of Medicine November 13, 1997; 337: 1419–1429.

Perricone, N., *The Wrinkle Cure: Unlock the Power of Cosmeceuticals for Supple, Youthful Skin*. Time Warner Book Group, New York, New York, 2000.

National Rosacea Society http://www.rosacea.org

Canadian Cancer Society. *Canadian Cancer Statistics 2005*. http://www.cancer.ca/vgn/images/portal/cit_86751114/48/2 8/401594768cw_2005stats_en.pdf

Wright, S., Burton, J.L., *Oral evening-primrose oil improves atopic eczema*. Lancet 1982; ii:1120–1122.

Perricone, N.V., *Photoprotective and Anti-Inflammatory Effects of Topical Ascorbyl Palmitate*. J. Ger Derm. 1993; 1: 5–10.

Packer, L. and Fuchs, J. (editors), *Vitamin C in Health and Disease*. Marcel Dekker, New York, 1997.

Fuchs, J., Packer, L. and Zimmer, G., *Lipoic Acid in Health and Disease*. Marcel Dekker, New York:, 1997.

Perricone, N.V., DiNardo, J.C., *The Photoprotective and Anti-Inflammatory Effects of Topical Glycolic Acid*. Derm Surgery, vol. 22 May1996; 5: 435–437

Hall, G. and Phillips, T.J., *Estrogen and skin: The effects of estrogen, menopause, and hormone replacement therapy on the skin*. J Am Acad Dermatol, October 2005: 555–565.

Chapter Six: Stress

Earle, R., Emrie, D., and Archbold, R., *Reduce Your Body Age: Clinically proven to reduce your body age by 11 years and restore youthful vitality!* The Canadian Institute of Stress, 1988.

Chapter Seven: Sleep

National Sleep Foundation, *2000 Omnibus Sleep in America Poll (OSAP)*. www.sleepfoundation.org/publications/2000 poll.html.

Sloan, E., Flint, A. and Shapiro, C., *Keeping Pace with Circadian Rhythm Problems in the Elderly*. The Canadian Journal of Diagnosis March 1994: 99–111.

Morris A. and Shapiro, C., *Insomnia in Older Adults. Part 1: Assessment*. Geriatrics And Aging vol. 7 July/August 2004; No 7: 3–8.

Swift, C. and Shapiro, C., *ABC of Sleep Disorders. Sleep and Sleep Problems in Elderly People*. British Medical Journal. 1993 May 29;306(6890):1468–71.

McAndrews, M.P., Weiss, R.T., Sandor, P. et al., *Cognitive Effects of Long-Term Benzodiazepine Use in Older Adults*. Hum Psychopharmacol of Clinl Exp. 2003; 18: 51–57.

National Highway Traffic Safety Administration and National Center on Sleep Disorders Research. *Drowsy Driving and Automobile Crashes: Report and recommendations*. DOT

Publication No. 808 707 April 1998, Washington, DC and Bethesda, MD.

National Sleep Foundation, *Facts about PLMS*. www.sleep-foundation.org/publications/fact-plms.html

Schneider, E., *The Longevity Quotient: calculate your odds of aging well and take steps now to stay youthful for life*. Rodale Inc. USA 2003.

Chapter Eight: Sex

Pfeiffer, E., Verwoerdt, A., Wang, H.S., *Sexual behavior in aged men and women*. Arch Gen Psychiatry 1968; 19(6):753–8.

Kaplan, H.S., *Sex, intimacy, and the aging process*. J Am Acad Psychoanal 1990; 18(2):185–205.

Meston, C.M., *Aging and sexuality*. West J Med 1997; 167(4): 285–90.

Crenshaw, T.L., Goldberg. J.P., *Sexual pharmacology: Drugs that affect sexual function*. New York W.W. Norton; 1996: 1–596.

Feldman, H.A., Goldstein, I., Hatzichristou, D.G. et al., *Impotence and its medical and psychosocial correlates: Results of the Massachusetts Male Aging Study*. J Urol 1994; 151(1): 54–61.

WebMD/Lycos Article, *Natural Menopause*. December 6, 2000. http://webmd.lycos.com/content/dmk/dmk_article_5963051

Sex and the Elderly. December 6, 2000 http://www.umkc.edu/sites/hsw/age/index.html

Byer, C., Shainberg, L., and Galliano, G., *Dimensions of Human Sexuality*. Boston: McGraw-Hill College 1999.

Courtenay, W.H., *Constructions of masculinity and their influence on men's well-being: A theory of gender and health*. Soc Sci Med 2000; 50(10): 1385–1401.

Nusbaum, M.R.H., Lenahan, P. and Sadovsky, R., *Sexual health in aging men and women: Addressing the physiologic and psychological sexual changes that occur with age.* Geriatrics. September 2005, vol. 6, No, 9.

Johannes et al., *Massachusetts Male Aging Study.* J. Urology 163: 460–463, 2000.

Sommers, F., *Visually Enhanced Psycho-Sexual Therapy (VEST) in a Multicultural Community.* The Canadian Journal of Psychiatry, December 2003, vol. 48, No. 11.

Sexual Health infoCenter. *Sex And Aging.* December 6, 2000. http://www.sexhealth.org/infocenter/SexAging/tips.htm

Chapter Nine: Memory

American Federation for Aging Research, *What Cognitive Changes Take Place With Age?* Neurobiology of Aging Information Center February 2004. http://www.infoaging.org/b-neuro-1-what.html

Bialystok, E., Viswanathan, M., Craik, F., Klein, R., *Bilingualism, Aging, and Cognitive Control: Evidence From the Simon Task.* Psychology and Aging, vol. 19, No. 2.

Morris, M. C., Evans, D. A., Bienias, J. L. et al., *Dietary Fats and the Risk of Incident Alzheimer Disease.* Arch Neurol. 2003; 60: 194–200.

Joseph, J. A., Shukitt-Hale, B., Denisova, N. A. et al., *Reversals of Age-Related Declines in Neuronal Signal Transduction, Cognitive, and Motor Behavioral Deficits with Blueberry, Spinach, or Strawberry Dietary Supplementation.* J. Neurosci, September 1999; 19: 8114–8121.

Morris, M. C., Evans, D. A., Bienias, J. L. et al., *Dietary Fats and the Risk of Incident Alzheimer Disease.* Rush Institute of Healthy Aging. *Arch Neurol.* 2003;60:194–200.

Anson, R. M., Guo, Z., de Cabo, R. et al., *Intermittent fasting dissociates beneficial effects of dietary restriction on glucose metabolism and neuronal resistance to injury from calorie intake*. PNAS 2003 100: 6216–6220.

Duan, W., Guo, Z., Jiang, H. et al., *Dietary restriction normalizes glucose metabolism and BDNF levels, slows disease progression, and increases survival in huntingtin mutant mice*. PNAS 2003 100: 2911–2916.

Mukamal, K. J., Kuller, L. H., Fitzpatrick, A. L. et al., *Prospective Study of Alcohol Consumption and Risk of Dementia in Older Adults*. JAMA, March 2003; 289: 1405–1413.

Snowdon, D. A., Greiner, L. H., Markesbery, W. R., *Linguistic ability in early life and the neuropathology of Alzheimer's disease and cerebrovascular disease: Findings from the Nun Study*. Journal of Personality and Social Psychology 2001; 80(5): 804–813.

Saczynski, J. S., Pfeifer, L. A., Esther, K. M. et al., *The Effect of Social Engagement on Incident Dementia: The Honolulu-Asia Aging Study*. Am J Epidemiol. 2006; 163:433–440.

MayoClinic.com. Tools for healthier lives. SENIOR HEALTH, *How to keep your mind sharp: Preventive action*. http://www.mayoclinic.com/health/memory-loss/HA00001

Levy, B., *Improving Memory in Old Age Through Implicit Self-Stereotyping*. Journal of Personality and Social Psychology. 71: 1092–1107, 1996.

Krieglstein, J., *Neuroprotective properties of Ginkgo biloba-constituents*. Zeitschrift Phytother 1994; 15:92–6.

Mix J.A., Crews W.D., *An examination of the efficacy of Ginkgo biloba extract EGb761 on the neuropsychologic functioning of cognitively intact older adults*. J Altern Complement Med 2000; 6:219–29.

Morris, M.C., Beckett, L.A., Scherr, P.A. et al., *Vitamin E and vitamin C supplement use and risk of incident Alzheimer disease.* Alzheimer Dis Assoc Disord 1998; 12:121–6.

Schmidt, R., Hayn, M., Reinhart, B. et al., *Plasma antioxidants and cognitive performance in middle-aged and older adults: results of the Austrian Stroke Prevention Study.* J Am Geriatr Soc 1998; 46:1407–10.

Masaki, K.H., Losonczy, K.G., Izmirlian, G. et al., *Association of vitamin E and C supplement use with cognitive function and dementia in elderly men.* Neurology 2000; 54:1265–72.

Imagawa, M., Naruse, S., Tsuji, S. et al., *Coenzyme Q10, iron, and vitamin B6 in genetically-confirmed Alzheimer's disease.* Lancet 1992; 340:671 [letter].

Meador, K., Loring, D., Nichols, M. et al., *Preliminary findings of high-dose thiamine in dementia of Alzheimer's type.* J Geriatr Psychiatry Neurol 1993; 6:222–9.

Blass, J.P., Gleason, P., Brush, D. et al., *Thiamine and Alzheimer's disease. A pilot study.* Arch Neurol 1988; 45:833–5.

Cervilla, J. A., Prince, Martin, Mann, Anthony, *Smoking, drinking, and incident cognitive impairment: a cohort community based study included in the Gospel Oak project* J Neurol Neurosurg Psychiatry May 2000; 68:622–626.

Chapter Ten: Mind, Body and Soul

Dembe, E., *Passionate Longevity: The 10 Secrets to Growing Younger.* John Wiley & Sons Canada Ltd., 2003.

Dembe, E., *Use the Good Dishes: Finding Joy in Everyday Life.* MacMillan Canada, 2000.

About the Authors

DR. PAUL COHEN

Board-certified dermatologist Dr. Paul Cohen is a clinical associate at Sunnybrook and Women's Health College Sciences Centre, and Fellow of the Royal College of Physicians and Surgeons of Canada. He has private offices in Toronto, Ontario.

An active member of, and key spokesman for, the Canadian Dermatology Association, Dr. Cohen has made over 80 television appearances on shows including Global News, Money Wise, Entertainment Tonight Canada, CBC news, CBC midday, CBC marketplace, Balance Television for Living Well and CTV news, as well as regular segments on Canada AM. He has been quoted in numerous publications such as the National Post, the Globe and Mail and the Toronto Star.

Dr. Cohen completed his medical training at the University of Toronto in 1995 and his dermatology training in Toronto in 2001. Awarded the Ben Fisher Galderma Fellowship in clinical dermatology, he then went on to complete fellowship training in pediatric and cosmetic dermatology.

DR. ELAINE DEMBE

Dr. Elaine Dembe's special kind of healing philosophy — "to touch the lives of others with my positive energy" — has helped thousands of patients to feel better physically and emotionally. An accomplished chiropractor of 28 years, she specializes in the care and prevention of back and neck problems, sports injuries and stress-related complaints.

A sought-after keynote speaker and media personality, she has given presentations to more than 300 leading corporations, associations and charitable organizations in Canada and the United States. Her irrepressible personality has won her the accolade of "cheerleader for life" and a designation as "the passion doctor." Dr. Dembe, who is also a life coach, has an extraordinary ability to focus on issues that block a person's path to health and wellness, inspiring people to reach their health potential.

Dr. Dembe is the author of two best-selling books: *Passionate Longevity: 10 Secrets to Growing Younger* (first edition 1995) and *Use the Good Dishes: Finding Joy in Everyday Life* (2000).

MIKE DEMETER

Mike Demeter has a Bachelor of Physical and Health Education from the University of Toronto with additional courses in nutrition sciences, psychology, naturopathic nutrition and strength and conditioning. With certifications in Fitness Appraisal from the Canadian Association of Sports Sciences and Muscle Testing from The Society of Weight Training Injury Specialists, Mike has enjoyed helping a diverse clientele with their various fitness and health aspirations. For several years he has been the Head Judge for the Canadian Federation of Fitness Competitions,

Recently he has applied his wealth of expertise to training stressed executives, a focus that has earned him a spot among Goodlife's Top Trainer of the Year finalists for five consecutive years.

DR. RICHARD EARLE

As Director of both the Canadian Institute of Stress and the Hans Selye Foundation, Dr. Richard Earle has continued to develop the research and educational commitments of his mentor and colleague, Dr. Hans Selye.

Prior to joining the Institute and the Foundation on a full time basis in 1982, Dr. Earle held senior consultative and program management posts with the governments of Canada and several of its provinces. His research focuses — stress and the biomarkers of human aging, and biopsy-chosocial factors in workplace change — have led to appointments to professional associations in North America, Europe and Japan.

He has held graduate faculty appointments in several universities since 1969, in departments Psychology, Sociology, Nursing and Medicine. Originating in 2002, his distance education of Certified Stress & Wellness Consultants has trained physicians, chiropractors plus related health and workplace specialists in North America, Europe and Japan.

Dr. Earle is senior author of *Reduce Your Body Age: Clinically proven to reduce your body age by 11 years and restore youthful vitality!*

To learn more about the Institute, please visit www.stresscanada.org

DR. THEODORE HERSH

Dr. Theodore Hersh (aka Dr. Ted) is an award-winning clinician, medical innovator and educator.

Dr. Ted received his undergraduate degree from Harvard University before attending medical school at Columbia University. He then went on to postgraduate training at Mount Sinai Hospital, the Mayo Clinic and Boston City Hospital. Upon graduation he spent two years in private practice in Mexico before returning to the U.S. to continue his career in research and academia at such esteemed institutions as Yale University, Baylor College of Medicine, Brown University and finally Emory University, where he served as Chairperson of Emory's Institutional Review Board for clinical research for 23 years.

Making all of these accomplishments even more amazing is the fact that Dr. Ted is almost completely blind. In 1980, he was diagnosed with Retinitis Pigmentosa, a progressive, degenerative eye condition that eventually forced him to retire from academia at age 62.

A few short years later he founded Thione International and, utilizing the eyesight of his wife Rebecca, began conducting antioxidant research. He currently has numerous patents and formulations under development.

DR. COLIN SHAPIRO

Dr. Colin Shapiro is Director of the Sleep Research Laboratory and of the Sleep & Alertness Clinic at Toronto Western Hospital, University Health Network, and a Fellow of The Royal College of Physicians and Surgeons of Canada.

Dr. Shapiro earned his undergraduate and MBBCh degrees in 1973 and 1977 respectively, from the University of the Witwatersrand in Johannesburg, South Africa. While a medical student he had the opportunity to study under Drs. William Dement and Christian Guilleminault, pioneers in modern sleep understanding. In 1985 he completed his PhD at the University of Edinburgh.

Dr. Shapiro's research in sleep and sleep disorders has led to numerous appointments nationally and abroad. More recently he has developed formal interests in providing information to both family physicians and the general public. The author of 15 books and more than 250 academic papers, Dr. Shapiro has appeared on numerous television and radio programs and is frequently referenced in newspaper and magazine articles. He currently serves as Senior Editor of the Journal of Psychosomatic Research and is a Professor in the Department of Psychiatry at University of Toronto.

DR. JOEY SHULMAN

One of North America's foremost authorities on nutrition and wellness, Dr. Joey Shulman is a highly sought-after speaker and writer, educating large audiences across North America about health and wellness.

No stranger to the media, Dr. Shulman makes frequent radio and television appearances on the Vicki Gabereau show, Canada AM, Cityline, the Discovery channel, CBC radio and television, the Women's network, Breakfast Television, CFRB 1010, MOJO radio and numerous other radio and television stations throughout Canada. A distinguished member of the General Advisory Board for Healthy Woman publications, she frequently contributes to several publications including Canadian Living, Homemakers, Healthy Woman magazine, mochasofa.com and Alive Magazine, and currently serves on the medical advisory board for Alive publications.

Dr. Shulman received a doctorate of chiropractic degree from the Canadian Memorial Chiropractic College and an honours degree in psychology from Concordia University. She is also a registered nutritional consulting practitioner (RNCP).

In addition to her duties as the vice-president of nutrition for Truestar Health, a leading online health site, Dr. Shulman is a health expert for genuine health supplements and head nutritionist for Sweetpea Baby Food, a line of top quality, frozen organic baby food.

Dr. Shulman is the author of *Winning the Food Fight: Every Parent's Guide to Raising a Healthy, Happy Child* (2003) and *The Natural Makeover Diet: A 4-Step Program to Looking and Feeling your Best from the Inside Out* (2006).

DR. FRANK SOMMERS

Frank G. Sommers, MD, FRCPC, is a psychiatrist specializing in the treatment of marital and sexual problems and currently is in private practice in Toronto.

Creator of the Great Sex video, an award-winning instructional film series on human sexuality, Dr. Sommers has pioneered research into applications of audio-visual media in the service of psycho-sexual therapy. Over the past 30 years he has authored a book and many articles and made frequent appearances on radio and television in Canada, the United States and Europe.

Dr. Sommers received his MD from the University of Toronto, where he continued on the teaching staff in the Department of Psychiatry. In addition, he is honorary and founding president of Canadian Physicians for Social Responsibility, and a Fellow of the Royal College of Physicians. Dr. Sommers' website is: www.drsommers.com

SHERRY TORKOS

Sherry Torkos is a pharmacist, author and certified fitness instructor. She received her Bachelor of Science degree in Pharmacy from the Philadelphia College of Pharmacy and Science in 1992, and practices in the Niagara region of Ontario.

A leading health expert, she has delivered hundreds of lectures to medical professionals and the public. She is frequently interviewed on radio and TV talk shows throughout North America, including Good Morning Canada, Help TV, The Perfect Fit and The Good Life Show.

In 1994, she was awarded the Commitment to Care Award for Providing Excellence in Patient Care from Pharmacy Practice magazine and, in 1999, the J.C. Gould Memorial Award for Distinguished Practice. Sherry has authored eight books, including *Winning at Weight Loss* (Wiley 2005), *The Benefits of Berries* (Bearing 2005), *Proven Natural Solutions for Depression* (Wiley, 2004), and *Breaking the Age Barrier* (Penguin Books, 2003).

DR. STEVEN YOUNG

Dr. Steven Young is a Certified Prosthodontist and Fellow of the Royal College of Dentists of Canada.

The descendant of a long line of dentists, including his father, brother, uncle, brother-in-law and several distant cousins, Dr. Young was literally born into dental care. In 1989 he earned his Doctor of Dental Medicine degree at Boston University and in 1992 completed his Hospital Residency and Certificate in Combined Prosthodontics at the State University of New York. Upon graduation he was awarded membership in Omicron Kappa Upsilon Honour Dental Society and began his existing teaching position as an Associate in Dentistry with the Department of Prosthodontics, Faculty of Dentistry, at University of Toronto.

Dr. Young is currently in private practice in Toronto and Mississauga.

DR. GORDON WINOCUR

Dr. Gordon Winocur is Vice President, Research at the Baycrest Centre for Geriatric Care and a Senior Scientist at the Rotman Research Institute. He is also Professor of Psychology and Psychiatry at the University of Toronto, and Professor of Psychology at Trent University.

Funded by the Canadian Institutes of Health Research, the Natural Sciences and Engineering Research Council of Canada and the J.F. McDonnell Foundation, Dr. Winocur's research is concerned with changes in memory and related cognitive function associated with normal aging, brain-damage and neurodegenerative disease. He has published over 150 articles in scientific journals, two books and 25 book chapters.

Dr. Winocur is a Fellow of the Canadian Psychological Association, American Psychological Association and the Association for Psychological Science. In addition to his research work, he is a frequent speaker at international conferences and has lectured at academic and clinical institutions in many countries around the world.